Success Probability
Estimation with Applications
to Clinical Trials

Success Probability Estimation with Applications to Clinical Trials

Daniele De Martini
Department of Statistics and Quantitative Methods
University of Milano-Bicocca
Milan, Italy

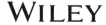

Library of Congress Cataloging-in-Publication Data:

De Martini, Daniele, 1965–
  Success probability estimation with applications to clinical trials / Daniele De Martini.
    p. ; cm.
  Includes bibliographical references and indexes.
  ISBN 978-1-118-33578-9 (cloth)
  I. Title.
  [DNLM: 1. Clinical Trials as Topic. 2. Probability. 3. Pharmaceutical Preparations. 4. Statistics as
Topic. QV 771.4]
  610.72'4—dc23   2013001310

Printed in the United States of America.

10 9 8 7 6 5 4 3 2 1

To my family

CONTENTS IN BRIEF

CONTENTS

PREFACE

This book aims to provide a simple and understandable introduction to the statistical techniques of success probability estimation.

Success probability estimation offers an original and practical perspective to the two problems: 1) evaluating the statistical significance and the stability of an experiment whose data analysis is based on a statistical test (e.g. a phase III trial), in order to avoid, if possible, further confirmatory studies; and 2) planning experiments on the basis of pilot data (e.g. phase III trials on the basis of phase II data), taking into account the variability of pilot data.

It is worth noting that these two problems have a common mathematical core, that is, the estimation of the true power of the test, namely the success probability. Usually, the power of statistical tests is viewed as a mathematical function, and it is studied analytically to compare these tests. Here, the new perspective is to estimate the true power of the tests, in other words, to estimate the success probability of experiments based on statistical tests.

The introduction, regarding clinical trials in general and reporting of some remarkable numbers related to them, opens the book. Then, the book is divided into two Parts: I) Success Probability Estimation in Planning and Analyzing Clinical Trials; and II) Success Probability Estimation for Some Widely Used Statistical Tests.

The first part presents the concepts related to success probability estimation and their usefulness in applied statistics, and in clinical trials in particular. Part I is devoted to both statisticians and non-statisticians (for example, clinicians who are involved in clinical trials).

The second part is mainly of interest to statisticians. An in depth analysis is provided on the techniques for success probability estimation, with applications both to reproducibility probability estimation and to conservative sample size estimation of some widely used statistical tests.

D. DE MARTINI

Genoa, Italy
March, 2013

ACKNOWLEDGMENTS

I would like to thank the *Department of Statistics* of *Stanford University*, where I visited several times, for the exceptional intellectual atmosphere I breathed there. I would also like to thank the *Department of Statistics and Quantitative Methods* (DiSMeQ) of the *Università degli Studi di Milano-Bicocca* for supporting this book.

With regards to single individuals, I wish to warmly thank Dr. Maurizio Rainisio and Dr. Lucio De Capitani, who revised the manuscript and gave me some useful suggestions.

D.D.M.

ACRONYMS

1SES	One Standard Error Strategy
3QS	Third Quartile Strategy
AN	Asymptotic Normality
AP	Average Power
BAS	Bayesian Strategy
BAT	Bayesian Truncated Strategy
COS	Calibrated Optimal Strategy
CSSE	Conservative Sample Size Estimation
dfs	Degrees of Freedom
edf	Empirical Distribution Function
iff	If and Only if
MC	Monte Carlo
MSE	Mean Square Error
OP	Overall Power
PWS	PointWise Strategy

RP	Reproducibility Probability
SP	Success Probability
SS	Single Study
SSE	Sample Size Estimation
WRS	Wilcoxon Rank-Sum

INTRODUCTION: CLINICAL TRIALS, SUCCESS RATES, AND SUCCESS PROBABILITY

This book considers experiments whose data are analyzed through statistical tests. A significant outcome of a test is considered a success, whereas a non-significant one is a failure.

Data are supposed to be collected with a certain amount of randomness, which implies the adoption of statistical tests for data analysis. Consequently, also the outcomes of the tests, i.e. success/failure, are affected by randomness. So, the probability of a successful outcome in these experiments, i.e. the probability of a significant outcome, is of great interest to researchers, sponsors of research and users of research results.

Focus is placed on large experiments that have been preceded by pilot ones. A pilot experiment is often performed in order to achieve data for deciding whether or not to launch the successive, important study and, if this is the case, to adequately plan the latter.

One of the contexts in which the framework above can be found is that of clinical trials. Here, large experiments are phase III trials, and previous phase II studies can be considered pilot studies in view of the subsequent phase III studies. A brief introduction to clinical trials follows, together with some data on their success rates and an introduction to their individual probability of success.

To conclude, in order to introduce applied problems related to success probability estimation, and to motivate the latter, two practical situations often encountered in clinical trials are presented, which can also be understood by those owning minimal statistical skills.

The context of clinical trials is adopted throughout the book to present, explain, and exemplify success probability estimation. Nevertheless, the fields of application of success probability estimation are numerous, and one example is that of quality control.

I.1   Overview of clinical trials

Clinical trials are implicit to drug development and are conducted to collect safety and efficacy data for health intervention. Clinical drug development is structured into four phases (see also the U.S. National Institute of Health - NIH; website: *clinicaltrials.gov*):

- Phase I trials include introductive investigations to study the metabolism and pharmacologic actions of drugs in humans, and the side effects associated with increasing doses. They are also run to furnish early evidence of effectiveness.

- Phase II trials are controlled studies conducted to evaluate the effectiveness of the drug for a particular indication in patients with the specific disease under study and to determine the common short-term side effects and risks.

- Phase III trials are expanded controlled studies that are performed once preliminary evidence suggesting effectiveness of the drug has been obtained. They are also intended to gather additional information on the overall benefit-risk relationship of the drug.

- Phase IV trials are post-marketing studies that are run to obtain additional information including the drug's risks, benefits, and optimal use.

In recent years, on average (approximately) 2600 phase I, 3700 phase II, 2300 phase III, and 1800 phase IV trials annually have been presented for approval under the United States Food and Drug Administration (FDA) (source: *clinicaltrials.gov*). These trials amount to about 60% of those run globally every year. Indeed, as a rule of thumb, the total amount of trials run worldwide is divided as follows: 60% under the United States Food and Drug Administration (FDA); 30% under the European Medicines Agency (EMA); and the remaining 10% under other Agencies, mainly the Japanese Pharmaceuticals and Medical Devices Agency (PMDA). It follows that an impressive number of trials are simultaneously in operation around the world every year.

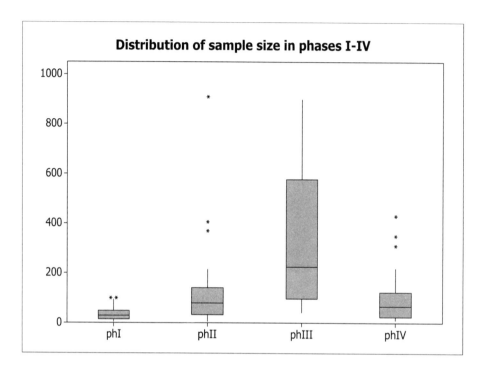

Figure I.1   *Sample size of clinical trials in different phases.*

The average size of the sample of patients enrolled in clinical trials varies considerably among the different phases. Also, within trials of the same phase the differences in sample size are very large. In order to have an idea of the order of magnitude of the sample sizes in different phases, the official U.S. NIH site of clinical trials was consulted, and a sample of year 2011 trials was drawn for each of the four phases (each sample of clinical trials was size 30). The sampling distributions of the sample size are illustrated in Figure I.1. Note that phase III trials are clearly the largest, while phase I trials are the smallest. To better understand the numbers, Table I.1 reports sampling averages and quartiles of sample size distributions.

It is evident that clinical trials involve a very large number of patients (and, in phase I, of healthy volunteers) every year, all over the world. Ethical concerns, therefore, arise. In fact, clinical trials have to be strictly evaluated by appropriate ethical committees.

Another important aspect to be considered in clinical trials is cost. Beside being high, in some circumstances even prohibitive for small companies, during the last

Table I.1   Sample size measures of the different clinical trial phases.

	Average	I quartile	Median	III quartile
Phase I	36	15	29	49
Phase II	128	33	80	141
Phase III	511	98	225	577
Phase IV	101	24	67	124

decade they have increased at a rate of about 4-5% per year. Some sources report an average cost per patient in phase I during 2011 of about $20000 and of about $30000, $40000 and $15000 (rounding down) in phases II-IV. The research and development costs of a new drug is estimated to be, as an order of magnitude, around U.S. $1 billion; some sources indicate that it recently grew to $1.3-1.7 billion. During 2011, more than $30 billion were spent on clinical research, in the United States alone.

Clinical trials may or may not succeed due to many factors, chiefly clinical, technological, or organizational. Of course, the eventual success is firstly due to the actual safety and efficacy of the drug under study. A relevant number of trials among the different phases of the drug development are not successful. In particular, the outcomes of the experiment do not reach the endpoints of safety and/or efficacy of the experimental protocol. Remarkably, the number of failures can also include trials whose experimented drug is actually safe and effective.

Success probability estimation techniques touch, in this context, ethics and economics and may help to improve the rate of success of clinical trials.

I.2   Success rates of clinical trials

The success rate of the population of clinical trials varies among the developmental phases, between the primary and secondary objectives of the trial (usually the lead indication presents a much higher rate of success), among therapeutic areas (for example, the success rate in oncology is usually lower than that in infectious diseases, and even among different oncological areas the rates are different), and among molecule type (where New Molecule Entities show a lower success rate than non-NME and biologic ones).

The success rates of the four phases of clinical research that are reported by different sources vary a bit. In Table I.2 the approximated success rates, averaged from various sources (FDA and EMA among others), are shown.

The final success rate of drugs, conditional to their success in phase I, is 19.2% (i.e. $80\% \times 60\% \times 40\%$). Analogously, the overall rate of success of drugs that enter phase I is 12.5% (actually, it goes from 9% to 15% among various sources).

Table I.2   Success rates of the different clinical trial phases.

	Unconditional Success Rate	Conditional Success Rate
Phase I	65%	12.5%
Phase II	40%	19.2%
Phase III	60%	48%
Phase IV	80%	80%

A number of factors influence the failure of clinical trials where clear evidence of therapeutic efficacy should be proved through the significance of statistical tests. Various sources indicate that in phase II and phase III trials, approximately 50% of failures are due to safety and clinical/strategic/organizational reasons (e.g. the dose administered is ineffective, the outcome measures used to determine drug effect are not sensitive enough to detect a change, the population considered may be inappropriate for proving effectiveness, or the new drug has a new mechanism of action). As a further consideration, note that approximately the same ates of failure of this kind, varying around 50%, are observed in all therapeutic areas.

The remaining 50% of failures is due to a lack of proved efficacy. Sometimes, the drug in question is actually not effective. Often, the efficacy shown is not high enough to be considered valid proof (this is also because failure is a lack of proved efficacy, not a lack of efficacy).

This 50% rate due to a lack of proved efficacy is astonishing. So, why do promising clinical trials fail? Often, *clinical trials fail just by chance*. Randomness is, indeed, one of the components of the experimental data to be analyzed, on which the outcome of success/failure of the trial, based on the result of the statistical test, depends. Consequently, even if the drug/compound is effective and safe, and the trial is based on a perfectly designed experiment, the trial does not succeed just by chance.

I.3 Success probability

The concept of *probability of success* of experiments (and in particular of clinical trials) stems from randomness. This implies that there exists a certain success probability (SP) for every single clinical trial. SP should not be confused with success rate: the latter refers to the population of clinical trials, whereas the former is peculiar to every single trial. Of course, SP is firstly due to the actual safety and efficacy of the drug under study and is more favorable when clinical and organizational errors are avoided in the experimental protocol.

The SP of a well planned experiment should be high, but not 100%. Indeed, the probability of failure of an *ideal* experiment (i.e. 100% minus SP) is usually 10-20%. This probability is the so-called type II error (see Chapters 1 and 3). This error exists because only infinite data assure that SP is 100% (this would imply no errors when the drug is effective), whereas in practice data are a finite number.

Moreover, it is not infrequent that a drug which has already succeeded in phase II, where effectiveness was proved, is actually ineffective, so that the subsequent phase III fails. This is due, once again, to randomness. The rate of these kinds of erroneous trials can be controlled since it coincides with the probability error allowed in the statistical significance of phase II, namely type I error (see Chapter 1). Usually, the latter error quantity is set at 5%-10%, but in some cases in phase II it may be even higher (see Chapter 3).

These type I and II errors concur in determining the 50% rate of failure of phase III trials reported in the previous Section. In order to compute how these errors actually weigh upon the failures, they should be jointly related to the 50% rate.

Suppose, for example, that the sum of type I error probability in phase II and of type II error probability in phase III is 20% - this is in agreement with the ranges of these errors reported above. Then, the failure rate due to these errors is given by the 50% of failures multiplied by the 20% of total error probability, and it results 10%. There still remains a 40% rate of failures (i.e. 50% minus 10%) depending on the lack of proved efficacy where the drug in study is actually effective, which is quite considerable.

Except for studies where the drug is actually ineffective (i.e. those under type I error), the SP depends on the amount of evidence that is planned to be collected to prove efficacy. In other words, SP depends on the size of the collected sample. This sample size is often based on predictions on the amplitude of the effect size of the drug in study. Various sources argue that these predictions are often too optimistic, causing several trial failures. These considerations should be related to the rate of unsuccessful trials whose drug under study is effective (i.e. 40% of the example above).

We can intervene on the latter set of trials to improve their peculiar SP through the study and, more importantly, the estimation of the SP itself. A practical problem to motivate SP estimation in relation to the amplitude of the sample size follows below (Section I.4.2).

Estimating the SP is also useful for successful experiments based on statistical tests, and not just for unsuccessful ones. Since the concept of *reproducibility* is a hinge of the scientific method, the estimation of the reproducibility probability (RP) of a successful experiment is a useful indicator of the stability of the outcome of the experiments, where RP is strictly related to SP. In the context of clinical trials, it is very useful to have an estimate of the RP on hand for the 60% of successful phase III trials (see Table I.2). This is also due to the regulatory agency requirements, as shown in the practical problem introducing RP estimation that follows in Section I.4.1.

I.4   Starting from practice

I.4.1   Situation I: reproducibility problems

A phase III large multicenter study to evaluate a new drug succeeded, providing significant results. The p-value of the two-tailed test was somewhat lower than the usual threshold of 5%, and it resulted 3%.

Regulatory agencies (such as the U.S. FDA and the European EMA) usually require a minimum of two significant studies to demonstrate the effectiveness of a new treatment. So, the question is: in order to reproduce a statistical significant result, is it correct to plan a further trial identical to the one above? And, in particular, what is the probability of reproducing the successful outcome? In other words: what is the probability of finding another p-value lower than 5% in a second, identical, confirmatory phase III trial?

Focusing on the planning of the second trial, should the sample size be the same as the experiment just performed, or, from a conservative perspective and in order to decrease the risk of a future non-significant result, should it be increased? An example dedicated to success probability and sample size problems is presented in the next Situation II, and answers to sample size questions will be provided in Chapters 3 and 4.

With regards to the probability of reproducing the observed successful outcome, how high is this quantity called RP? Should the significant observed outcome be considered a fortunate one? For example, if it is assumed that the data observed in the study reproduce exactly the population behavior (e.g. the sample means coincide with the population ones) the reproducibility probability is just about 58%. So, this successful outcome can actually be viewed as a fortunate one.

Now, assume that the observed p-value was 1%. Regulatory agencies sometimes allow the omittance of the second confirmatory pivotal trial, provided that statistically very persuasive findings are shown (more details on this point can be found in Chapter 2). So, can this outcome be considered persuasive enough to be sufficient for approval without one or more confirmations? What about the variability of the data? The latter variability generates consequent variability in the outcomes of statistical tests (i.e. in statistical significance) and can therefore provide non-significant outcomes in further studies. In other words, is the statistical significance of the latter outcome *stable* enough, even when the variability of the data is taken into account? For instance, is the observed 1% p-value, with respect to the statistical significance threshold of 5%, estimated to be reproducible enough? How high is its reproducibility probability estimated to be? Can a conservative estimate for the latter quantity be computed?

Reproducibility probability estimation will be studied in Chapter 2, and the questions above will be answered at the end of it.

I.4.2 Situation II: sample size problems

In a phase II trial, two groups of 59 patients each were compared in order to demonstrate the superiority of a new drug, and the experiment did provide promising results. In particular, considering the effect size to be the standardized difference between the two means (i.e. $(\mu_1 - \mu_2)/\sigma$), an estimate of the effect size of 0.48 was observed. This value was considered of clinical relevance, since the threshold of minimum scientific relevance for the effect size was considered to be 0.15. Also, statistical significance at the threshold of 5% was found, and the p-value was about 1%. As a consequence, the research team decided that the subsequent phase III trial was to be launched and adequate planning would, therefore, be necessitated.

On this basis, how many subjects should be enrolled in order to have a probability of a 90% success? In other words, how large should the sample size be in order to plan a phase III trial with a 90% probability of success?

Let's consider the effect size as 0.48, then the traditional and simple computation of the sample size provides a sample size of 92 patients per group. But, would this be the right solution?

Of course, the desired 90% probability of success will not result unless luck is involved: there might be, in fact, very different probabilities of success, varying, for example, from 99.8% to a considerably worse 38.0% one! Indeed, what about the variability of the $59 + 59$ phase II data giving the *estimated* effect size of 0.48? It must be remembered that this effect size is, in fact, just an estimate that may be more or less close to the unknown, true, effect size. Every estimate allows for a certain range of plausible values, and in this case they range (around 0.48) from 0.244 to 0.716 (i.e. the bounds of an 80% confidence interval with $n = 59$ data per group). And, the latter effect size values (i.e. the lower and the upper bounds of the effect size) actually result in a success probability of 38.0% and 99.8% with 92 data per group.

Taking this into consideration, some practical questions arise: should the whole range of plausible values be considered, or just the observed one, provided that the latter is of clinical relevance? If the observed effect size is considered, then the probability that this is higher than the unknown effect size is 50%; consequently, the actual probability of success is lower than 90% half of the time: is this rate too risky? In order to reduce this 50% rate, would it be sufficient to consider a conservative modification of the observed effect size?

If, for example, instead of the point estimate 0.48, 75% is considered to be the amount of conservativeness of the estimate of the effect size (i.e. the lower bound of a 50% confidence interval), which results 0.3558, on one hand the estimated sample size would increase to 166 data per group, but on the other hand a strategy would have been adopted that reduces the probability to plan an underpowered experiment to $1/4$. Would this conservative approach be better than the simplest one, i.e. the one adopting the observed effect size?

In practice, when the variability of the effect size is taken into account, different strategies for computing the sample size arise, potentially providing very different values. So, what are the differences among their performances and, more importantly, which sample size estimation strategy is the best?

In Chapter 3 these concerns will be discussed, and answers to these questions will be provided. Moreover, in Chapter 4 further situations will be discussed, such as those where the effect size of the new drug in phase II may be different from that of the subsequent phase III.

PART I

SUCCESS PROBABILITY ESTIMATION IN PLANNING AND ANALYZING CLINICAL TRIALS

The first part of the book presents the concepts related to success probability estimation and their usefulness in clinical trials. Part I is devoted to both statisticians and non-statisticians: each Section of the first four Chapters begins with a boxed text explaining, in non-technical and non-statistical language, the concepts contained in the Section.

Chapter 1 illustrates the basic statistical tools and introduces the success probability (SP). In Chapter 2 the SP of a new trial with identical settings of the one previously performed is studied; this probability assumes the meaning of reproducibility probability (RP). The evaluation of the stability of the results of statistical tests is presented, together with the important new tool of RP-testing, which allows statistical testing only on the basis of the estimate of the RP. In Chapter 3 the use of pilot data for estimating SP and then the sample size of a subsequent trial is studied. In other words, the problem of planning clinical trials on the basis of pilot samples is discussed. The important concepts of launching criteria are introduced, and the

Success Probability Estimation with Applications to Clinical Trials, First Edition.
By Daniele De Martini Copyright © 2013 John Wiley & Sons, Inc.

variability of pilot data is taken into account, leading to the so-called conservative sample size estimation (CSSE). Several CSSE strategies are introduced and their performances are compared. In Chapter 4 the robustness of CSSE strategies is evaluated, and some correction techniques are presented and compared.

In order to present SP estimation techniques and their application, in this first Part the statistical test for comparing the means of two Gaussian distributions with known common variances will be adopted. The first population represents patients under a new drug, the second one includes those under a control treatment. In order to facilitate the reader, samples of equal sizes are assumed to be drawn from the two populations; this will be the same throughout Part I. Generalization concerning different sample sizes will be developed in Part II, as well as techniques for SP estimation of other statistical tests.

CHAPTER 1

BASIC STATISTICAL TOOLS

This Chapter provides some basic statistical concepts and tools. Pointwise estimation and confidence interval estimation are introduced; conservative estimation follows. Then, an explanation is given on what statistical tests are. The power function of the tests together with the errors of first and second type are defined. The p-value is presented, as an index for evaluating the outcome of the test. Some applications in the context of clinical trials are shown and numerical examples and figures are also provided. The probability of success in a trial (i.e. success probability) is illustrated, including how to estimate it. Superiority tests are adopted first to illustrate the above topics. Then, inequality tests are considered. Finally, there is a brief Section regarding how success probability estimation can be derived for tests of clinical superiority, of non-inferiority and for equality tests.

Success Probability Estimation with Applications to Clinical Trials, First Edition.
By Daniele De Martini Copyright © 2013 John Wiley & Sons, Inc.

1.1 Pointwise estimation

Two populations are in the study, representing tho one treated with a new drug and that treated with a control drug. In order to estimate the unknown parameters of interest of these populations, for example their averages (i.e. means), experimental samples are drawn from the populations. Then, experimental data are used to provide an estimated value, which is often the most likely one, of these parameters: this is *pointwise estimation*.

Often, the effect size of the new drug is the quantity of clinical interest and is expressed as the ratio of the difference between the two means and the common standard deviation of the distributions. So, the effect size can be estimated on the basis of point estimates of means and standard deviation derived from population samples. It is worth noting that the frequency of effect size estimates that are far from the true (and unknown) value of the effect size tends to be smaller as the size of the samples tends to be larger.

Nevertheless, although the point estimate is probably close to the unknown effect size, especially for large samples, it is almost surely different from the true effect size. What is most important is that pointwise estimation has its peculiar *random variation*, since it depends on random samples. Estimates, indeed, can vary from one sample to another and they vary randomly since samples are randomly drawn. Consequently, the variability of pointwise estimates must be taken into account during the estimation process. This is a very basic and essential statistical concept.

Consider two Gaussian distributions representing the distributions of the quantity of interest in the two patient populations being treated with the new drug (population 1) and with the control (population 2), defined by X_1 and X_2, respectively. These distributions have generic means μ' and μ'', respectively, and common standard deviation σ. This σ is a measure of the variability of population data around their means - it is a mean of the distances of data from the respective means.

The *effect size* of the experiment is considered here to be the standardized difference between the means, that is $\delta = (\mu' - \mu'')/\sigma$. The effect size can cover a wide range of values, depending on how the new and the control drugs perform. Nonetheless, there is only one "true" value of δ, namely δ_t and given by the true means μ_1 and μ_2. To investigate on δ_t is the aim of our research.

A sample of size m is randomly drawn from each patient population and the random variables representing the data provided by the patients are denoted by $X_{i,j}$, with $j = 1, \ldots, m$ and $i = 1, 2$. The sample averages $\sum_{j=1}^{m} X_{i,j}/m$, denoted by $\bar{X}_{i,m}$, aim to estimate the distribution means μ_i, $i = 1, 2$, and are *estimators* of the latter. Since estimators are functions of the random samples they are random variables too. In general, estimators are built in order to fall with high probability close to the parameters they are estimating.

Here, σ is assumed to be known. The pointwise estimator of δ_t is, then, based on sample averages: $d_m = (\bar{X}_{1,m} - \bar{X}_{2,m})/\sigma$.

The value that a random variable assumes, i.e. the observed value of the latter, is called *realization* of the random variable; the realizations of estimators are called *estimates*.

Remark 1.1. *Often, distinct notations are adopted to emphasize the difference between a random variable and its realization: uppercase and lowercase letters usually indicate the former and the latter object, respectively. For example, the realizations of the average of the first sample (i.e. the estimates of μ_1) might be denoted by $\bar{x}_{1,m}$. Throughout the book, this distinction will not be made and the reader will deduce from the context of the sentence if either a random variable or a realization of it is being considered.*

■ **EXAMPLE 1.1**

The variables X_1 and X_2 of the two populations under study have true mean $\mu_1 = 5$ and $\mu_2 = 1$, respectively, and standard deviation $\sigma = 8$. The shape of their Gaussian distributions is shown in Figure 1.1. The true effect size, therefore, is $\delta_t = (5-1)/8 = 0.5$. A sample of size $m = 85$ is drawn from each population, providing the estimates $\bar{X}_{1,85} = 3.816$ and $\bar{X}_{2,85} = 1.152$ (these are realizations of $\bar{X}_{1,85}$ and $\bar{X}_{1,85}$). It is not surprising that sample mean estimates do not coincide with population ones: this is due to random variation. The effect size estimate is $d_{85} = (3.816 - 1.152)/8 = 0.333$.

Without loss of generality, and in order to handle as few symbols as possible, σ is set equal to 1 throughout Part I of this book, whenever not explicitly claimed, the contrary. Then, $\delta_t = \mu_1 - \mu_2$. Consequently the pointwise estimator of the effect size, which is a function of the estimators of the unknown parameters, is:

$$d_m = \bar{X}_{1,m} - \bar{X}_{2,m} \tag{1.1}$$

The probability distribution of d_m, as a consequence of the Gaussian distribution shapes of the populations, is Gaussian too - this is due to a mathematical theorem. The mean of d_m is δ_t, and its standard deviation is $\sigma_{d_m} = \sigma\sqrt{2/m}$, which is also called the *standard error* of d_m; being $\sigma = 1$, we have $\sigma_{d_m} = \sqrt{2/m}$. This means that d_m is more dense around δ_t, and that the probability that d_m falls far from δ_t decreases, as the sample size m increases. In other words, the precision in estimating δ_t improves when m increases (see Figure 1.2). Formally speaking, d_m is a *consistent* estimator of δ_t. Recall that d_m is a random quantity, depending on random samples, and that its realizations vary from one couple of samples to another.

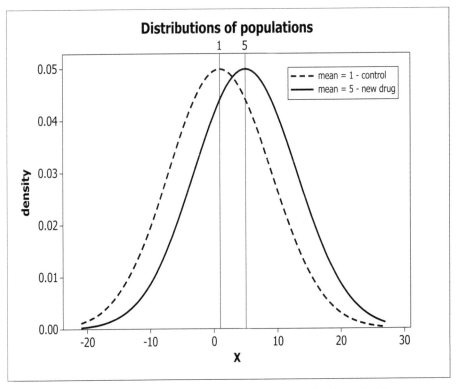

Figure 1.1   *Distributions of the populations in study - Example 1.1.*

1.2   Confidence interval estimation, conservative estimation

The variability of pointwise estimates is here taken into account. Indeed, beside the point estimate, an interval of admissible value for the unknown quantity of interest (in this case, the effect size) should be provided. This interval, too, is based on random samples, and so it may or may not include the effect size.

The key concept is that the probability that the so-called *Confidence Interval* contains the true effect size can be controlled. This probability, namely *confidence level* of the interval (viz. γ), is usually set high (e.g. $90 - 95\%$). Its complement to 1 (i.e. $1 - \gamma$) is the error probability, i.e. the probability that the Confidence Interval does not contain the true effect size.

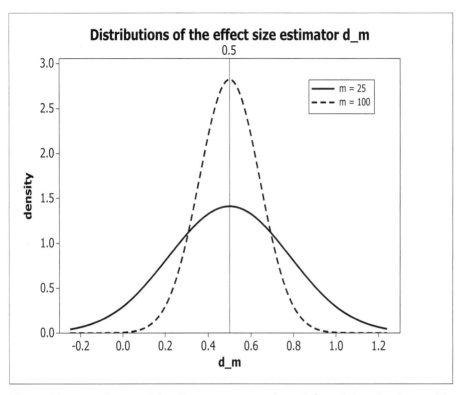

Figure 1.2 *Distributions of the effect size estimator d_m with $\delta_t = 0.5$, and with $m = 25$ and 100. It is of note that the distribution of d_{100} is more dense around $\delta_t = 0.5$ than that of d_{25}.*

Note that as the sample sizes increase the amplitude of the interval decreases, so that confidence interval estimation becomes more precise. On the contrary, the probability of error does not change with the sample sizes.

The lower bound of the confidence interval can be viewed as a conservative estimate of the effect size: it tends to the latter as the sample size increases, remaining below it with a given (high) probability.

In order to derive an interval of plausible values for δ_t (namely Confidence Interval) the standardized version of d_m is introduced, that is $(d_m - \delta_t)/\sqrt{2/m} = \sqrt{m/2}(d_m - \delta_t)$. The latter quantity has a Gaussian distribution with mean 0 and variance 1, namely a standard Gaussian distribution.

A random variable with the latter distribution is represented by the symbol Z. The terms Gaussian distribution and normal distribution will be used as synonyms.

Now, let Φ be the cumulative distribution function of the standard normal, that is the probability that Z falls below a certain value t: $\Phi(t) = P(Z \leq t)$). Moreover, let z_γ be the γ-th percentile of the standard normal (i.e. z_γ is such that $P(Z \leq z_\gamma) = \gamma$). Then, the γ-percentile is $z_\gamma = \Phi^{-1}(\gamma)$.

It follows that the central part of the distribution of Z lies, with probability γ, in the interval $[z_{(1-\gamma)/2}, z_{(1+\gamma)/2}]$. Since the standardized version of d_m is Z-distributed, we obtain:

$$P(z_{(1-\gamma)/2} \leq \sqrt{m/2}(d_m - \delta_t)/ \leq z_{(1+\gamma)/2}) = \gamma$$

Inverting the two inequalities above, and being $z_{1-\gamma} = -z_\gamma$ due to the symmetry of the Gaussian distributions, we finally have:

$$P(d_m - z_{(1+\gamma)/2}\sqrt{2/m} \leq \delta_t \leq d_m + z_{(1+\gamma)/2}\sqrt{2/m}) = \gamma \qquad (1.2)$$

In other words, the (random) interval $[d_m - z_{(1+\gamma)/2}\sqrt{2/m}, d_m + z_{(1+\gamma)/2}\sqrt{2/m}]$ contains δ_t with probability γ, and so it is a γ-Confidence Interval for the effect size. This is a two-sided confidence interval, since it is both upward and downward bounded. The confidence level γ is usually set high, e.g. $90\%, 95\%, 99\%$.

■ **EXAMPLE 1.2**

Let us continue Example 1.1, where the effect size estimate was $d_{85} = 0.333$. With a confidence level $\gamma = 95\%$, $z_{(1+\gamma)/2}$ becomes $z_{97.5\%} = 1.96$ (see Table A.1). The realizations of the bounds of the interval result: $0.333 - 1.96\sqrt{2/85} = 0.032$ and $0.333 + 1.96\sqrt{2/85} = 0.634$. In this case, the realization of the interval contains $\delta_t = 0.5$.

Note that the confidence interval is defined by a random quantity (i.e. d_m) and so it varies from one couple of samples to another. γ is the frequency of sampled confidence intervals that contain δ_t, independently on m. The amplitude of the interval is given by the difference between its upper and lower bounds and it results $2z_{(1+\gamma)/2}\sqrt{2/m}$, which decreases as m increases. This means that confidence interval estimation improves its precision as the sample size increases. The confidence level γ does not change when m varies.

Confidence Intervals can also be one-sided. In fact, when a statistical lower bound for the effect size is of interest, the one-sided γ-Confidence Interval is:

$$[d_m - z_\gamma\sqrt{2/m}, +\infty)$$

which provides:

$$P(d_m - z_\gamma\sqrt{2/m} \leq \delta_t) = \gamma \qquad (1.3)$$

The lower bound of the interval can be used for *conservative estimation*. Being:

$$d_m^\gamma = d_m - z_\gamma \sqrt{2/m} \qquad (1.4)$$

the latter can be viewed as a conservative estimator of the effect size In other words, d_m^γ tends to be much closer to δ_t as the size of the sample m increases, with the condition of falling below δ_t with (high) probability γ (see Figure 1.3). Let us call d_m^γ the γ-*lower bound for* δ_t.

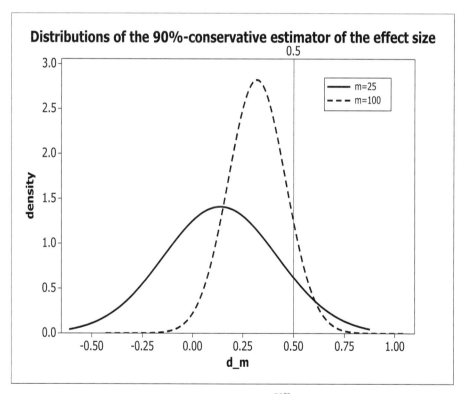

Figure 1.3   *Distributions of the effect size estimator $d_m^{90\%}$ with $\delta_t = 0.5$, and with $m = 25$ and 100. It is of note that $d_{100}^{90\%}$ is more dense around $\delta_t = 0.5$ than $d_{25}^{90\%}$, and that the area under the curves below 0.5 equals 90% (i.e. the amount of conservativeness of $d_m^{90\%}$) for each m.*

1.3 The statistical hypotheses, the statistical test and the type I error for one-tailed tests

The statistical test is the procedure that leads, through the statistical analysis of experimental data, to one of these two outcomes: "it is experimentally proved that the new drug is more effective than the control drug", or "it is not proved that the new drug is more effective". The possibility to prove that the new drug is less effective than the control treatment will be considered later.

In practice, the assumption that the mean of the effect of the new drug is lower than, or at least equal to, that of the control drug is made. In other words, it is assumed that the true effect size is lower than, or equal to, zero, viz. *null hypothesis*. If clinical trial data show, under the latter assumption, an unexpected result, that the patients respond considerably better under the new drug, then the assumption above (against the new drug) is rejected, the complementary assumption (i.e. the true effect size is greater than zero, viz. *alternative hypothesis*) is assumed to be true, and the effectiveness of the new drug is considered to be experimentally proved.

Specifically, a sample of patients is randomly drawn from each population and the respective sample means are computed. Hence, if a high difference is observed in favor of the new drug, so high that this observed event falls within the predefined set of events having globally, under the null hypothesis, a low probability (namely α), then the statement "it is experimentally proved that the new drug is more effective than the control drug" is the outcome of the test - this is called a *significant* outcome. Otherwise, the outcome is "it is not proved that the new drug is more effective", and nothing is proved.

In case the drug is considered to be effective where in actual fact it is not, an error is made: this is the type I error of the test. The probability that this error occurs is at most α. This α is set before recruiting patients, and so before analyzing data, it is often equal to 5% or to 2.5%.

The assumptions on the means are the *statistical hypotheses*, which formally result in:
$$H_0 : \mu_1 \leq \mu_2 \qquad \text{and} \qquad H_1 : \mu_1 > \mu_2$$
namely the *null* and the *alternative* hypotheses, respectively. The latter is the one-sided alternative of *superiority*. Further hypotheses (such as $H_1 : \mu_1 > \mu_2 + \delta_0$) will be considered later (see Section 1.8) . Note that the hypotheses can also be viewed in terms of effect size:
$$H_0 : \delta_t \leq 0 \qquad \text{and} \qquad H_1 : \delta_t > 0$$

The test statistic, namely T_m, has to reflect the behavior of the phenomenon of interest and is, therefore, a function of the samples of size m drawn from the two populations. Here, the difference between the means is under study, and so T_m is built on the basis of sample averages, and in particular of d_m. Moreover, d_m is divided by its standard deviation σ_{d_m}, so that T_m has a unitary standard deviation:

$$T_m = (\bar{X}_{1,m} - \bar{X}_{2,m})/\sigma_{d_m} = d_m/\sqrt{2/m} = \sqrt{m/2}\,d_m \qquad (1.5)$$

T_m has a Gaussian distribution with mean $\delta_t \sqrt{m/2}$ and variance 1 - see Figure 1.4. (When the null hypothesis is $H_0 : \mu_1 \leq \mu_2 + \delta_0$, i.e. $H_0 : \delta_t \leq \delta_0$, then $d_m - \delta_0$ is considered so that $T_m = \sqrt{m/2}(d_m - \delta_0)$ - see Section 1.8). Under the null hypothesis, T_m has mean at most 0.

It follows that large values of T_m could lead one to consider it true that $\delta_t > 0$ (or that $\delta_t > \delta_0$ when $H_1 : \mu_1 > \mu_2 + \delta_0$ is under testing) and induce H_0 rejection.

Then, the probability, namely α, permitted to the type I error, i.e. rejecting H_0 when it is true, is set. So, the rejection region, i.e. the set of values that if assumed by T_m induce H_0 rejection, is that on the right tail of the standard Gaussian distribution whose total probability is α, that is $(z_{1-\alpha}, +\infty)$. In other words, the null hypothesis is rejected when T_m results greater than $z_{1-\alpha}$, which is named the *critical value of the test*. Note that the probability to reject H_0 when it is true is actually, at most, α: $P_{\delta_t=0}(T_m > z_{1-\alpha}) = \alpha$.

The statistical test ψ_α, therefore, is:

$$\psi_\alpha(T_m) = \begin{cases} 1 & \text{if} \quad T_m > z_{1-\alpha} \\ 0 & \text{if} \quad T_m \leq z_{1-\alpha} \end{cases} \qquad (1.6)$$

where "1" stands for "H_1 is experimentally proved" and "0" for "nothing is proved".

This ψ_α is also called Z-test. Here, the rejection region is defined on one tail of the distribution of the test statistic under the null, and so ψ_α is named *one-tailed* test.

1.4 The power function and the type II error

The power function of the test reports the probability to reject the null hypothesis, that is the probability to prove that the new drug is more effective than the control drug. This probability depends on the type I error, on the sample size and on the generic effect size δ.

When the null hypothesis is true, the power function, i.e. the probability to reject the null, provides the probability of an error: this is the type I error, whose probability assumes at most the value of α.

When the alternative hypothesis is true, that is when the new drug is effective, there is actually the possibility of not rejecting the null hypothesis. If this happens an error is made: this is the type II error, whose probability is named β and is given by 1 minus the power function.

Table 1.1   Errors and Right Decisions (RD), with their probabilities, in hypotheses testing.

	Hypotheses	
Decisions	H_0 true	H_1 true
Accept H_0	RD	type II error
	$1 - \alpha$	β
Reject H_0	type I error	RD
	α	$\pi(\alpha, m, \delta)$

Consider now a generic value δ of the effect size, not the fixed and unique true effect size δ_t. Then, the generic test statistic T_m is normally distributed with mean $\delta\sqrt{m/2}$ (not $\delta_t\sqrt{m/2}$) and unitary variance. From (1.6) the probability to reject H_0 is $P_\delta(\psi_\alpha(T_m) = 1)$, i.e. $P_\delta(T_m > z_{1-\alpha})$. The latter quantity depends on α, m and δ and it is called the power function: $\pi(\alpha, m, \delta)$.

From the knowledge of the distribution of T_m we have:

$$\pi(\alpha, m, \delta) = P_\delta(T_m > z_{1-\alpha}) = P_\delta(T_m - \delta\sqrt{m/2} > z_{1-\alpha} - \delta\sqrt{m/2})$$

$$= P(Z > z_{1-\alpha} - \delta\sqrt{m/2}) = \Phi(\delta\sqrt{m/2} - z_{1-\alpha}) \tag{1.7}$$

Note that under H_0 (i.e. with values of $\delta \leq 0$) the power function is lower than, or equal to, the type I error:

$$\pi(\alpha, m, \delta) \leq \pi(\alpha, m, 0) = \Phi(-z_{1-\alpha}) = \Phi(z_\alpha) = \alpha$$

Given α and m, the power function (1.7) increases as δ increases, meaning that the probability to prove that $\delta > 0$ grows as the effect size becomes higher. The power function also increases, given α and $\delta > 0$, as the available information grows, that is as m increases. To complete, given m and δ, the power function is higher for larger αs.

Under the alternative hypothesis (i.e. with $\delta > 0$) a possible error could be to fail to reject H_0 - this is often called "to accept H_0". This is the type II error, whose probability is $\beta = 1 - \pi(\alpha, m, \delta)$. Under H_1, the power function (1.7) is higher than the type I error: $\pi(\alpha, m, \delta) > \alpha$ if $\delta > 0$. In Table 1.1 the possible decisions are summarized, together with their respective errors.

Remark 1.2. *It is noteworthy that to accept H_0 signifies that there is not enough information to reject it, and therefore to prove H_1. To accept H_0 does not mean,* *therefore, that the null hypothesis is proved: the null hypothesis is never proved. On the contrary, when H_0 is rejected H_1 is experimentally proved, unless the type I error is made, this probability is α.*

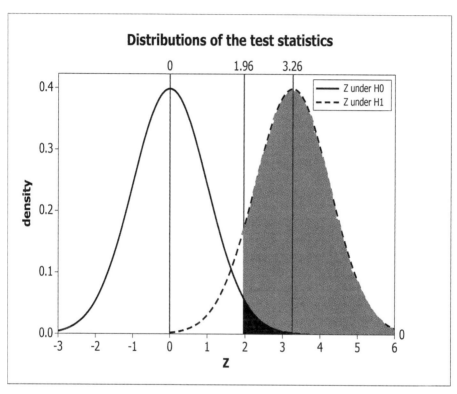

Figure 1.4 *Distributions of the test statistic under the null and under the alternative of Example 1.3 with $m = 85$. Note that the mean of T_{85} is $\delta_t\sqrt{m/2} = 0.5\sqrt{85/2} = 3.26$. The probabilities are represented by the area under the curves: the black area represents the type I error probability $\alpha = 2.5\%$ under the null; the gray-dashed area (which includes the black one) represents the probability, under the alternative, to fall in the rejection region with $m = 85$ and $\delta = 0.5$, that is $\approx 90\%$.*

▉ EXAMPLE 1.3

When $\alpha = 2.5\%$ the critical value is $z_{97.5\%} = 1.96$ (use Table A.1 to obtain probabilities and deviates for the standard normal distribution, and so even for power computation). When $\delta = 0.5$ the power function with $m = 17, 40$ and 85 data per group provides 30.78%, 60.88% and 90.31%, respectively, according *to (1.7). This means that with $m = 85$ available data, there is approximately a 90% probability to prove that $\mu_1 > \mu_2$, allowing for a type I error of 2.5%. In Figure 1.4 this 90.31% power can be viewed as a probability (the label Z is adopted for values of T_m, as in the next Figures). The power functions are reported in Figure 1.5.*

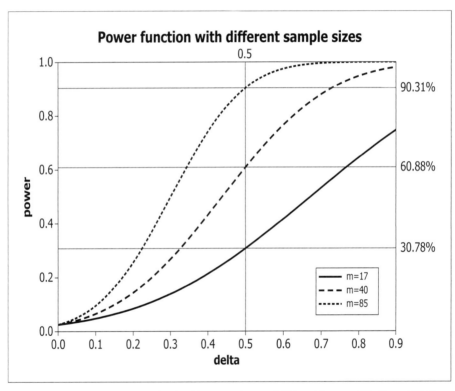

Figure 1.5   *Power functions for the Z-test with $\alpha = 2.5\%$, with $m = 17, 40$ and 85 (i.e. for scenarios in Example 1.3). The values assumed by the power functions with $\delta = 0.5$ are reported.*

1.5   The p-value

> The p-value is the statistical index traditionally used for evaluating the outcome of statistical tests: given the data, the p-value is the maximum type I error for which a test statistic is not significant.
>
> Another possible way to introduce the p-value is that it represents the probability, computed under the null hypothesis, of finding, in a new experiment completely analogous to that just performed but independent of it, a result even farther from the null hypothesis than the one just observed.
>
> In other words, the p-value answers this question: if the null hypothesis is really true (in this case, if $\delta_t \leq 0$), what is the probability that random sampling would lead to a result better than the one observed in favor of the new drug (e.g. a difference between sample means larger than the one observed)?
>
> The p-value is an index of the strength adopted to reject the null hypothesis: the lower than α the p-value is, the higher the strength.
>
> Moreover, the p-value can also be used to compute the outcome of the test: the null hypothesis is, indeed, rejected only when the p-value results lower than the prefixed type I error probability α.

Let us define the p-value formally:

$$\text{p-value} \quad = \quad \max\left\{\alpha' \text{ s.t. } \psi_{\alpha'}(T_m) = 0\right\} \tag{1.8}$$

From the test statistic (1.6) and the definition (1.8), the p-value is such that $T_m = z_{1-\text{p-value}}$. Then, recalling the definition of $z_x = \Phi^{-1}(x)$ and applying the monotone function Φ to both members of the latter equality we obtain:

$$\Phi(T_m) = \Phi(\Phi^{-1}(1 - \text{p-value})) = 1 - \text{p-value}$$

giving, finally:

$$\text{p-value} = 1 - \Phi(T_m) \tag{1.9}$$

Alternatively, the p-value can be defined by considering a new experiment, identical to the one just performed, which gives a new test statistic T_m^* independent of T_m. Hence, the p-value, being the probability under H_0 that the random statistic T_m^* would be larger than the observed T_m, can be defined as follows:

$$\text{p-value} = P_{\delta_t=0}(T_m^* > T_m \,|T_m) = 1 - \Phi(T_m)$$

where the last equality follows from the condition that the test new statistic T_m^* is Gaussian distributed, as in this introductory testing situation. (The notation $P(A|B)$ means "the probability of A once event B has been observed".)

■ **EXAMPLE 1.4**

Consider a one-tailed Z-test with type I error probability $\alpha = 2.5\%$, so that the critical value is $z_{97.5\%} = 1.96$. A total of 170 patients are recruited, and they are randomized into two groups of size 85. The latter represent the two samples from the two populations under the new drug and under the control treatment, providing sample averages of $\bar{X}_{1,85} = 0.477$ and $\bar{X}_{2,85} = 0.144$, respectively. From 1.5, the observed test statistic is: $T_{85} = \sqrt{85/2}(0.477 - 0.144) = 2.17$. Since T_{85} is greater than 1.96, the test outcome is significant: $\psi_{2.5\%}(2.17) = 1$. According to (1.9) the p-value is $1 - \Phi^{-1}(2.17) = 1.5\%$, which seems quite a bit lower than α (use Table A.1 also to compute p-values). Consequently, this outcome appears quite a reassuring one. The p-value is reported as a black area in Figure 2.1.

It is interesting to note that the p-value in (1.9) is lower than α only when T_m is over the critical value of the test, that is only when the outcome of the test is significant. Indeed, we have that:

$$\text{p-value} = 1 - \Phi(T_m) < \alpha \quad \text{iff} \quad \Phi(T_m) > 1 - \alpha \quad \text{iff} \quad T_m > \Phi^{-1}(1 - \alpha) = z_{1-\alpha},$$

where iff means *If and Only if*. So, the p-value can also be employed to define the statistical test (1.6) itself:

$$\psi_\alpha(T_m) = \begin{cases} 1 & \text{if} \quad \text{p-value} < \alpha \\ 0 & \text{if} \quad \text{p-value} \geq \alpha \end{cases} \qquad (1.10)$$

Equation (1.10) may be referred to as *p-value testing*.

As a consequence, the power function (1.7) (i.e. the probability of finding a significant outcome) can be viewed as the probability of finding a p-value lower than the type I error probability α:

$$\pi(\alpha, m, \delta) = P_\delta(T_m > z_{1-\alpha}) = P_\delta(\text{p-value} < \alpha)$$

Since the p-value depends on data, it is a random variable with a certain distribution. In Figure 1.6 the distributions of the p-value in scenarios of Example 1.3 are reported. Note that p-value distributions under the alternatives are much denser to the left for high power values, i.e. for high values of m. Moreover, when $\delta = 0$ (i.e. for the highest of the possible values under H_0) the p-value is uniformly distributed in $(0, 1)$, that is $P_{\delta_t = 0}(\text{p-value} \leq t) = t$, with $t \in (0, 1)$. In other words, in this case the density of the p-value is uniformly equal to 1 in the domain $(0, 1)$.

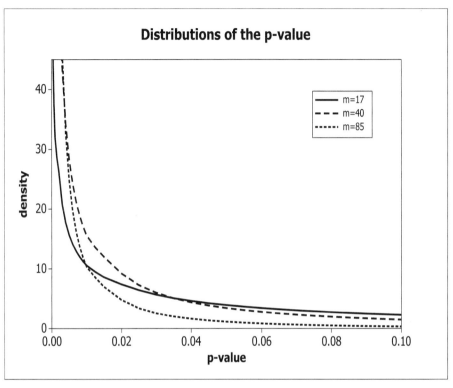

Figure 1.6 *Distributions of the p-value for the Z-test with $\alpha = 2.5\%$, under the alternative hypothesis with $\delta = 0.5$, $m = 17$, 40 and 85 (i.e. for scenarios in Example 1.3).*

1.6 The success probability and its estimation

The true probability of proving that the new drug is more effective than the control drug when it actually is, that is, the true probability of rejecting the null hypothesis under the alternative, is called the success probability, SP.

SP depends on the "true" value of the effect size, which is actually unknown. Of course, SP is related to the power function: in particular, SP *is* the power function evaluated at δ_t, when $\delta_t > 0$.

Since δ_t is unknown, the same holds true for SP. Nevertheless, it would be very useful to acquire information on SP, that can in fact be estimated.

SP estimation can be applied in solving the problems presented in Section I.4. In particular, it can be applied for estimating the sample size of a phase III trial on the basis of phase II data, and for estimating, once a trial has been performed, the probability of finding a statistical significance in a new trial whose settings are identical to those of the one just performed (namely *reproducibility probability*), in order to evaluate the *stability* of the results of the trial.

The SP is the power function computed at δ_t, that is:

$$SP = P_{\delta_t}(T_m > z_{1-\alpha}) = \pi(\alpha, m, \delta_t) = \Phi(\delta_t \sqrt{m/2} - z_{1-\alpha}) \qquad (1.11)$$

In other words, SP is the true power of the test.

Now, let us assume that two samples of size n (not necessarily equal to m) are available from the same two populations, one from each. (Actually, in Chapter 3, Section 3.2, it will be explained that the condition of sampling from the same populations can be relaxed). These samples can be viewed as pilot ones and are independent from those of size m used to define the Z-test in (1.6). On the basis of these data an estimator of δ_t can be computed: let us call it $d_n^{\bullet}$, where $\bullet$ indicates that several statistical approaches can be adopted for estimating δ_t (the simplest one is $d_n^{\bullet} = d_n = \bar{X}_{1,n} - \bar{X}_{2,n}$). Hence, an estimator of the SP is obtained by putting the estimator of δ_t in the power function definition (1.7):

$$\hat{SP} = P_{d_n^{\bullet}}(T_m > z_{1-\alpha} \mid d_n^{\bullet}) = \pi(\alpha, m, d_n^{\bullet}) = \Phi(d_n^{\bullet} \sqrt{m/2} - z_{1-\alpha}) \qquad (1.12)$$

This statistical practice of substituting an estimator of a parameter into a certain function of the parameter itself is called the "plug-in principle".

■ **EXAMPLE 1.5**

Consider the same sample data of Example 1.4. The observed effect size is $d_{85} = 0.477 - 0.144 = 0.333$ (as in Example 1.1) and it is considered the estimate of δ_t. Assume that it is of interest to estimate the SP of a one-tailed Z-test with $\alpha = 2.5\%$ enrolling $m = 120$ data per group (here 85 plays the role of n). From (1.12) the estimate of the latter quantity resulted: $\hat{SP} = P_{0.333}(T_{120} > z_{97.5\%}) = \Phi(\sqrt{120/2}\,0.333 - 1.96) = 73.22\%$. According to Example 1.1, where $\delta_t = 0.5$, $SP = P_{0.5}(T_{120} > z_{97.5\%}) = 97.21\%$. The power function with $m = 120$ is reported in Figure 1.7, together with SP and $\hat{SP}$.

SP estimation can be applied to solve the problems presented in Situations I and II of Section I.4.

Actually, Situation I considered a particular case of SP estimation, where the size of the test sample (i.e. m) is equal to that of a sample actually available, n. The SP estimation assumes, therefore, the meaning of *reproducibility probability* estimation. This topic will be developed in Chapter 2.

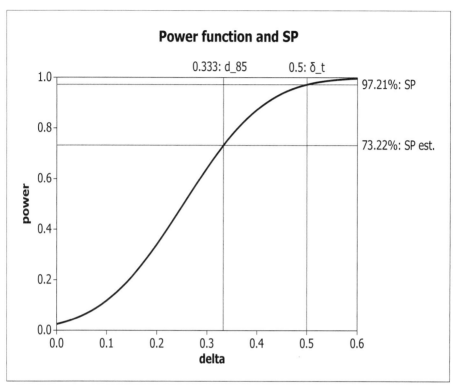

Figure 1.7 *Power function, SP and estimated SP for the Z-test with $\alpha = 2.5\%$, with $m = 120$, illustrating Example 1.5.*

Situation II concerned *sample size estimation*: in practice the sample size for a phase III can be computed on the basis of SP estimates given by phase II data. Different approaches to SP estimation are available, and they will be developed in Chapters 3 and 4.

1.7 Basic statistical tools for two-tailed tests

In this Section the basic statistical tools and SP definition will be extended to the two-tailed setting.

1.7.1 Two-sided hypotheses and two-tailed statistical test

When the statistical test procedure should provide one of these two statements: "it is experimentally proved that one of the drugs is more effective than the other one", or "it is not proved that neither drug is more effective", two-sided hypotheses are to be adopted.

The possibility that the new drug is less effective than the control treatment is included here. In other words, the assumption of *inequality* is being proved, instead of that of superiority.

In practice, the assumption that there is no difference between the means (i.e. the true effect size is zero, viz. *null hypothesis*) is made. If clinical trial data show a "strange" result, that is, a considerably better patient response to any of the drugs, then the assumption of no difference is rejected and the effectiveness of the drug which performed better is considered as experimentally proved.

Specifically, a sample of patients is randomly drawn from each population and the respective sample means are computed. If a high difference is observed, high enough that this observed event falls within the predefined set of events having globally, under the null hypothesis, a low probability α, then the first statement is the outcome of the test. Otherwise, the outcome is the second statement: nothing is proved.

The concept of type I error is analogous to that of Section 1.3: in case one of the drugs is considered to be more effective when actually it is not, an error is made, namely type I error of the test.

When two-sided alternatives are considered the statistical hypotheses under testing are:

$$H_0 : \mu_1 = \mu_2 \qquad \text{and} \qquad H_1 : \mu_1 \neq \mu_2$$

(one can also state $H_0 : \delta_t = 0$ and $H_1 : \delta_t \neq 0$). The latter H_1 is the two-sided alternative of *inequality*. The test statistic T_m is the same as the one defined in (1.5). Low values of T_m lead to infer that $\delta_t < 0$, and high values that $\delta_t > 0$, so that in both cases H_0 rejection is a probable outcome.

Under the null, T_m has a standard normal distribution. The probability allowed to the type I error, i.e. rejecting H_0 when it is true, is still α. So, the rejection region, i.e. the set of values that if assumed by T_m induce H_0 rejection, should consider both tails of the standard Gaussian distribution and α is, therefore, shared between the two tails, so that each part of the rejection region has $\alpha/2$ probability. Consequently, the null hypothesis is rejected when T_m results lower than $z_{\alpha/2}$ or greater than $z_{1-\alpha/2}$. The rejection region is, therefore, $(-\infty, z_{\alpha/2}) \cup (z_{1-\alpha/2}, +\infty)$. Note that the type I probability remains α: $P_{\delta_t=0}(T_m < z_{\alpha/2} \text{ or } T_m > z_{1-\alpha/2}) = P_{\delta_t=0}(T_m < z_{\alpha/2}) + P_{\delta_t=0}(T_m > z_{1-\alpha/2}) = \alpha/2 + \alpha/2 = \alpha$.

The statistical test ψ_α, therefore, is:

$$\psi_\alpha(T_m) = \begin{cases} 1 & \text{if} \quad T_m < z_{\alpha/2} \text{ or } T_m > z_{1-\alpha/2} \\ 0 & \text{if} \quad z_{\alpha/2} \le T_m \le z_{1-\alpha/2} \end{cases} \tag{1.13}$$

This test, where the rejection region is the union of two regions, one on each tail of the distribution of the test statistic under the null, is named *two-tailed* test.

1.7.2 Two-tailed power function, type II and III errors and SP

The power function reports the probability to reject the null hypothesis, that is the probability to prove that any of the drugs is effective. In this two-tailed context too, this probability depends on the type I error, on the sample size and on the generic effect size δ.

When the null hypothesis is true, the power function (i.e. the probability to reject H_0) coincides with the probability of the type I error, i.e. α.

When the alternative hypothesis is true, that is, when any of the drugs is more effective and null hypothesis is not rejected, an error is made: this is the type II error, whose probability (i.e. β) is 1 minus the power function (like in the one-tailed setting).

In case the alternative hypothesis is true and the null hypothesis is rejected but the worst drug is actually considered to be the best one, an error is committed: this is the type III error. The probability of the type III error is, in practice, very small and it can, therefore, be ignored.

In two-sided hypotheses testing, the SP is the probability to prove that any of the drugs is effective when one of the two is actually so (i.e. when $\delta_t \ne 0$), *avoiding the type III error*. This probability depends on the "true" value of the effect size δ_t, which is actually unknown. Even this two-tailed SP can be estimated.

In the two-tailed setting there are two possible significant outcomes (one for each tail of the null distribution) and so the power function of the test is the sum of the two following quantities:

$$\pi_2(\alpha, m, \delta) = P_\delta(T_m < z_{\alpha/2}) + P_\delta(T_m > z_{1-\alpha/2}) \tag{1.14}$$

We call these two summands $\pi_L(\alpha/2, m, \delta)$ and $\pi_R(\alpha/2, m, \delta)$ respectively, to indicate the probability to fall on the Left tail (i.e. below $z_{\alpha/2}$) and on the Right tail (over $z_{1-\alpha/2}$).

When $\delta \ne 0$ and the test fails to reject H_0 the type II error is made, whose probability is $\beta = 1 - \pi_2(\alpha, m, \delta)$. As for one-tailed tests, under the alternative the power function (1.14) is higher than the type I error: $\pi_2(\alpha, m, \delta) > \alpha$ if $\delta \ne 0$.

The type III error (Harter, 1957) consists in rejecting the null hypothesis and in deciding that the worst drug is the best one. Hence, under H_1, one of the two summands of the power function above (viz. $\pi_L(\alpha/2, m, \delta)$, $\pi_R(\alpha/2, m, \delta)$) is the probability of the type III error, and the other one can be viewed as the "good power function". Often, the type III error probability is very small and it always is lower than $\alpha/2$.

■ EXAMPLE 1.6

The values assumed by the type III error probability are often very small. For example, when $\alpha = 5\%$, if $\delta = 0.5 > 0$ and $m = 17$, the type III error probability is $\pi_L(2.5\%, 17, 0.5) = P_{0.5}(T_{17} < z_{2.5\%}) = 0.0316\%$. If δ decreases to 0.2 then the probability of the type III error increases to 0.55%. With $m = 40$ these two latter probabilities are 0.0014% and 0.22%, respectively, and they become even lower when m grows.

Now, let us define the SP on the basis of (1.14) and in accordance with its one-tailed definition (1.11). Note that the "good power function" is one of the two summands of (1.14), but which of the two is unknown. So, the SP for the two-tailed setting is the "good power function" evaluated at δ_t under the alternative hypothesis:

$$SP_2 = \begin{cases} P_{\delta_t}(T_m < z_{\alpha/2}) & \text{if} \quad \delta_t < 0 \\ P_{\delta_t}(T_m > z_{1-\alpha/2}) & \text{if} \quad \delta_t > 0 \end{cases} \qquad (1.15)$$

SP estimation for two-tailed tests will be developed later (see Sections 2.9 and 3.10).

1.7.3 Two-tailed p-value

The concept of the p-value has not changed: it remains, therefore, the maximum type I error for which a test statistic is not significant.

Here, the p-value answers this question: if the null hypothesis is really true (in this case, if $\delta_t = 0$), what is the probability that random sampling in a new experiment completely analogous to that just performed would lead to a difference between sample means larger than that observed, *in favor of each of the drugs?*

Even in this case the null hypothesis is rejected only when the p-value is lower than α.

The formal definition of the p-value in (1.8) is still valid, and through (1.13) gives:

$$\text{p-value} = 2(1 - \Phi(|T_m|)) \qquad (1.16)$$

In analogy with the one-tailed setting, the p-value can also be defined by considering the probability, under the null hypothesis, that a test statistic T_m^* given by a new experiment identical to the one just performed would be farther from 0, potentially in both directions/tails, than the observed T_m. This reflects in:

$$\text{p-value} = 2P_{\delta_t=0}(T_m^* > |T_m| \, | T_m) = 2(1 - \Phi(|T_m|))$$

In practice, the p-value is two times the probability mass, computed under the null, of the tail delimited by the observed test statistic. In other words, if, for example, $T_m > 0$ then the p-value is $2P_{\delta_t=0}(T_m^* > T_m \, | T_m) = 2(1 - \Phi(T_m))$.

Finally, the p-value based definition of the statistical test (1.10), i.e. p-value testing, remains valid.

1.8   Other statistical hypotheses and tests

In some circumstances, the statement "the new drug is more effective than the control" is related to a clinical minimum threshold of improvement. This concept introduces statistical tests of *clinical superiority*.

In other occasions different assumptions should be proved, such as "the new drug is as effective as a standard therapy". When this statement is related to a clinical maximum threshold of worsening of the new drug with respect to the standard therapy, this approach introduces statistical tests of *clinical non-inferiority*.

Further, *equivalence* statistical tests consider the simultaneous experimental proof of clinical non-superiority and clinical non-inferiority.

For all these tests, statistical analysis and SP estimation can be performed in analogy with those shown in previous Sections of this Chapter.

Let us consider a threshold of minimum clinical improvement $\delta_0 > 0$. It is interesting to prove the one-sided alternative of *superiority* $H_1 : \mu_1 > \mu_2 + \delta_0$, where the null hypothesis is $H_0 : \mu_1 \leq \mu_2 + \delta_0$. For these hypotheses the test statistic (1.5) becomes:

$$T_m = \sqrt{m/2}(\bar{X}_{1,m} - \bar{X}_{2,m} - \delta_0)$$

and the test of clinical superiority is defined as the test in (1.6).

Now, let $\delta_0 > 0$ be the threshold of maximum clinical worsening. Thus, the one-sided alternative of *non-inferiority* to be proved is $H_1 : \mu_1 > \mu_2 - \delta_0$, being $H_0 : \mu_1 \leq \mu_2 - \delta_0$. The test statistic, therefore, is:

$$T_m = \sqrt{m/2}(\bar{X}_{1,m} - \bar{X}_{2,m} + \delta_0)$$

and the test of clinical non-inferiority is once again equal to (1.6).

When $\delta_0 > 0$ represents the threshold of *clinical equivalence*, the alternative hypothesis of non-inferiority *and* non-superiority to be proved is $H_1 : |\mu_1 - \mu_2| < \delta_0$, that is $H_1 : \mu_2 - \delta_0 < \mu_1 < \mu_2 + \delta_0$. Complementarily, the null hypothesis of no equivalence is $H_0 : \mu_1 \leq \mu_2 - \delta_0 \cup \mu_1 \geq \mu_2 + \delta_0$. In this context, when the set representing H_0 is not convex, the statistical test is significant when $\sqrt{m/2}(\bar{X}_{1,m} - \bar{X}_{2,m} + \delta_0) > z_{1-\alpha}$ and $\sqrt{m/2}(\bar{X}_{1,m} - \bar{X}_{2,m} - \delta_0) < -z_{1-\alpha}$.

For clinical superiority and clinical non-inferiority tests, the SP is defined as in (1.11). In particular, for superiority tests the δ_t in (1.11) should be replaced by $\delta_t - \delta_0$, and for non-inferiority tests by $\delta_t + \delta_0$. The SP for equivalence tests can be obtained analogously, but this topic is not developed here.

CHAPTER 2

REPRODUCIBILITY PROBABILITY ESTIMATION

Scientific Method hinges on the reproducibility of experimental outcomes.

Clinical trials data are analyzed through statistical tests and, consequently, the reproducibility of their outcomes becomes relevant. Nevertheless, the outcomes of statistical tests, besides belonging to the set: {significant, non-significant}, are random ones because they depend on the sample(s) selected randomly and/or on the randomized allocation of the treatments. Hence, even the reproducibility of the test result inherits this randomness, and it should be evaluated in terms of probability of reproducing a certain outcome of the statistical test itself.

It is of note that a significant outcome represents experimental proof that the new drug is effective, whereas a non-significant one implies that nothing is proved. So, the quantity of main interest is the reproducibility probability of a statistically significant outcome in a new experiment, whose settings are identical to those of the old one. Nevertheless, since a non-significant result is not experimental proof of the null hypothesis and it may represent a type II error, it is assumed that the *reproducibility probability* (RP) is the probability of finding a significant outcome in a second experiment (with identical settings) *independently from the outcome of the first one*. RP is strictly related to success probability SP, and it is, indeed, a particular case of the SP.

Success Probability Estimation with Applications to Clinical Trials, First Edition.
By Daniele De Martini Copyright © 2013 John Wiley & Sons, Inc.

In this Chapter, the estimation of RP is first illustrated, stemming from the SP of the one-tailed setting. Then, the adoption of the estimate of RP to directly perform statistical tests is introduced - this technique is called RP-testing. Since the estimate of the RP represents an alternative indicator to the p-value, the relationships between these two quantities are shown. Moreover, the variability of RP estimates is taken into account: the technique for computing a confidence interval for RP is shown, leading to the evaluation of the *stability* of statistical test outcomes.

Some statistical criteria for stability are shown and compared, most of which are based on RP estimation. The point of view of regulatory agencies (viz. FDA, EMA) on the possibility of performing one single pivotal study (instead of the usual minimum of two) is shown, and it is discussed in relation with the stability criteria. All these concepts are also illustrated in a specific section for the two-tailed setting. To conclude, the application of RP estimation techniques to the introductive Situation I of Section I.4.1 is shown.

2.1   Pointwise RP estimation

SP is the true probability of finding a statistically significant result in a certain trial.

Assume that two samples are available from the two populations in study and that they undergo a statistical test.

Then, the SP of a trial based on samples of sizes equal to those available can be viewed as the SP of the ongoing trial or of any new completely analogous reproduction of the experiment. Hence the SP assumes the meaning of *reproducibility probability* (RP).

The RP depends on the type I error probability α, and so its estimate will be denoted by $\hat{RP}_\alpha$.

It is intuitive that $\hat{RP}_\alpha$ is useful to interpret the results of statistical tests: the more reproducible the outcome of the test, the more "stable" the outcome itself. Besides the p-value, $\hat{RP}_\alpha$ remains another index for evaluating the outcomes of statistical tests.

It should also be noted that the p-value, besides being criticized because of its not immediate understanding, might often lead to too optimistic interpretations of the test results in terms of reproducibility.

The SP, in a trial with m (potential, i.e. not yet recruited) experimental units per group, was $P_{\delta_t}(T_m > z_{1-\alpha})$ (see (1.11)).

When a sample of size n is available from each of the two populations in study, the SP with n data becomes, according to (1.11), $SP = \pi(\alpha, n, \delta_t)$, The latter SP can be viewed as the probability of finding a statistically significant outcome in the ongoing trial or in any new identical *reproduction* of the experiment. The true power $\pi(\alpha, n, \delta_t)$ can, therefore, be viewed as the *reproducibility probability* (RP).

Now, recall that T_n^* is the test statistic of a hypothetical future experiment: $T_n^* = \sqrt{n/2}(\bar{X}_{1,n}^* - \bar{X}_{2,n}^*)$, where $\bar{X}_{1,n}^*$ and $\bar{X}_{2,n}^*$ are the sample means of the two populations of the new experiment. Being $d_n^\bullet$ the generic estimator of the effect size δ_t, the estimator of RP of an experiment, based on the two n-sized samples, is $\pi(\alpha, n, d_n^\bullet) = P_{d_n^\bullet}(T_n^* > z_{1-\alpha})$. This quantity is an estimator of RP, whether or not the pilot experiment provides statistical significance (i.e. whatever $T_n > z_{1-\alpha}$ or not).

If the simple pointwise estimator of the effect size is considered (viz. $d_n^\bullet = d_n = \bar{X}_{1,n} - \bar{X}_{2,n}$), then the plug-in based RP estimator, in accordance with (1.12), becomes:

$$\hat{RP}_\alpha = P_{d_n}(T_n^* > z_{1-\alpha} \,|\, T_n) = \Phi(d_n\sqrt{n/2} - z_{1-\alpha}) = \Phi(T_n - z_{1-\alpha}) \quad (2.1)$$

In other words, the SP in a new identical trial, where the new effect size is estimated on the basis of $\bar{X}_{1,n}$ and $\bar{X}_{2,n}$, is computed. Note that the notation emphasizes the dependence of RP on α.

▦ EXAMPLE 2.1

Let us continue Example 1.4, where the sample averages of the two populations were 0.477 and 0.144, respectively, with $n = 85$ data per group. α was 2.5% and the p-value resulted 1.5%. The effect size δ_t is estimated to be $d_{85} = 0.477 - 0.144 = 0.333$. Assuming this value as the true one (i.e. that the estimate gives exactly the estimated parameter), the mean of the new test statistic T_{85}^* is $\sqrt{85/2} \times 0.333 = 2.17$. Consequently, the probability of finding a statistically significant outcome in a new experiment, computed through (2.1), is $\hat{RP}_{2.5\%} = P_{0.333}(T_{85}^* > z_{97.5\%}) = \Phi(2.17 - 1.96) = 58.3\%$ (see Table B.4 in Appendix B). To visualize probability computations, see Figure 2.1.

It is worth noting that, although the p-value appeared quite reassuring (1.5% seems not close to 2.5%), the RP estimate provides a worrying value: a 58.3% probability of reproducing a p-value lower than α is almost like a "dropping a coin" experiment! Actually, if the observed effect size is the true one, the observed positive outcome should be considered a fortunate one, since the probability of accepting H_0, i.e. of committing a type II error, is 41.7%.

The use of RP estimation was introduced by Goodman (1992). Making use of numerical examples like the above one, he argued that if the effect size observed in the study is the true one, then RP is substantially lower than that expected from observing the p-value. Ottenbacher (1996) provided an in-depth discussion on the concepts related to the replications of research findings and complained that randomness of statistical test outcomes is too seldom taken into account.

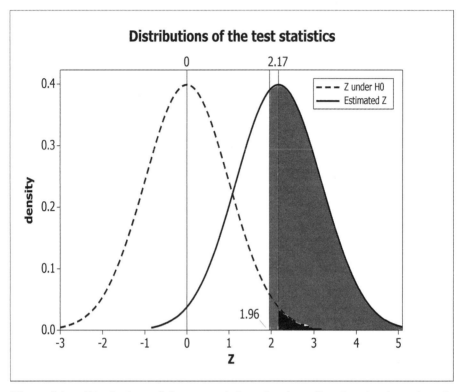

Figure 2.1   *Distributions of the test statistic under the null and under the estimated alternative of Examples 1.4 and 2.1: the black area represents the p-value of 1.5%; the gray area, which includes the black one, represents the estimated RP of 58.3%.*

▣ EXAMPLE 2.2

Continuing Example 2.1. Assuming that the sample average of the first population was 0.341 (instead of 0.477), the estimated effect size was $d_{85} = 0.341 - 0.144 = 0.197$. Then, the test statistic would be $T_{85} = \sqrt{85/2} \times 0.197 = 1.28$ (i.e. lower than the critical value $z_{97.5} = 1.96$) and consequently the test would not be significant. The p-value, indeed, would be 10% (use (1.9) and Table A.1). In this case, the RP estimate would be $\hat{RP}_{2.5\%} = P_{0.197}(T_{85}^{*} > z_{97.5\%}) = \Phi(1.28 - 1.96) = 24.9\%$ (once again, use (2.1) and Table B.4).

RP estimators are random variables, and therefore their distributions are of interest. Since p-values distributions have already been shown (Figure 1.6), the distributions of $\hat{RP}_{2.5\%}$ are now reported in Figure 2.2 for the same scenarios of Example 1.3

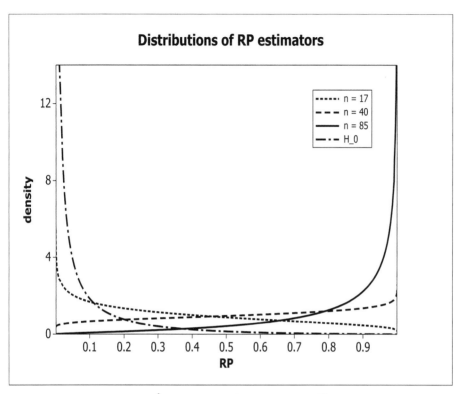

Figure 2.2 *Distributions of $\hat{R}P_{2.5\%}$ for the Z-test with $\alpha = 2.5\%$, under the null and under the alternative with $\delta_t = 0.5$, $n = 17$, 40 and 85 (scenarios of Example 1.3).*

(i.e. $\delta_t = 0.5$, $m = 17$, 40 and 85) and under the null. Note that under the null RP is denser to the left with a thin tail on the right. Under the alternative, as the sample size (and so the power) increases, the RP distributions become much denser to the right.

2.2 RP-testing

The statistical test can be defined directly on the sole basis of the estimate of the RP, that is $\hat{R}P_{\alpha}$. The threshold for the statistical significance of $\hat{R}P_{\alpha}$ is $1/2$.

In practice, H_0 is rejected and H_1 is experimentally proved when it is estimated that there is a higher probability of finding a significant outcome (i.e. of succeeding in proving H_1) than a probability of finding a non-significant one. Viceversa, H_0 is accepted when it is estimated that there is a higher probability of finding a non-significant outcome than a significant one. In other words,

the null hypothesis H_0 is rejected when it is estimated that there is a higher probability of rejecting it than accepting it.

This technique is called RP-testing. Hence, the RP estimate is not only an index of "stability" of test results, but can be actually adopted for defining the test itself, as does the p-value.

Note that in Examples 2.1 and 2.2, when a significant outcome of the test occurred, RP was estimated to be higher than $1/2$, whereas in a non-significant outcome it resulted lower. This is a general rule, independent of α and n: the test is significant if and only if the RP estimate is higher than $1/2$.

In particular, thanks to the definition of $\hat{RP}_\alpha$ in (2.1), we have that:

$$\hat{RP}_\alpha = \Phi(T_n - z_{1-\alpha}) > 1/2 \quad \text{iff} \quad T_n - z_{1-\alpha} > \Phi^{-1}(1/2) = 0 \quad \text{iff} \quad T_n > z_{1-\alpha}$$

Consequently, the test can even be defined on the basis of the RP estimator:

$$\psi_\alpha(T_n) = \begin{cases} 1 & \text{if} \quad \hat{RP}_\alpha > 1/2 \\ 0 & \text{if} \quad \hat{RP}_\alpha \leq 1/2 \end{cases} \tag{2.2}$$

Figure 2.1 is useful in the visualization of this result. Figure 2.3 is even more clear, reporting RP estimates and the threshold of $1/2$.

Besides equations (1.6) and (1.10) (i.e. the definitions of the statistical test based on acceptance/rejection regions and on the p-value, respectively), equation (2.2) represents the third way to define the test. Consequently, the outcome of the test can be read by looking directly for the RP estimate, without evaluating if the test statistic falls above the critical value, or if the p-value is lower than α. This technique for testing statistical hypotheses solely based on the RP estimator with threshold at $1/2$, which we recently introduced (see De Martini, 2008), is called *RP-testing*.

As will be shown in Chapters 5-9, RP-testing holds not only for the Z-test but can also be expanded to encompass many other statistical tests.

In particular, when data follow normal distributions, RP-testing can be applied to: the statistical tests for comparing two means with unknown variances, in the case of two-sample parallel designs as well as with crossover designs, where the test statistic has a Student's t distribution; the statistical test for the population variance, where the test statistic has a chi-square (i.e. χ^2) distribution; the statistical tests for comparing more than two means, and the one to compare the variances of two populations, where the test statistic has a Fisher F distribution.

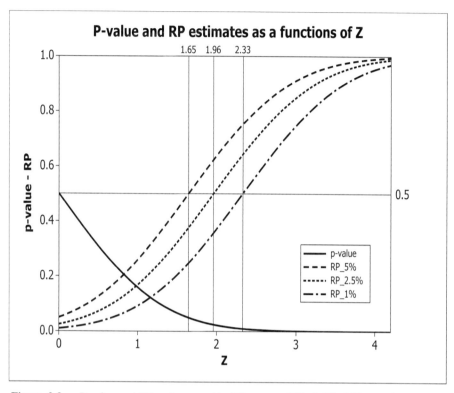

Figure 2.3   *P-value and RP estimates with different αs (5%, 2.5%, 1%) as a function of the test statistic, for the Z-test. Note that $\hat{RP}_\alpha$ is higher than its threshold of statistical significance (i.e. 0.5) iff the test statistic Z is higher than its threshold of significance $z_{1-\alpha}$ (i.e. 1.65, 1.96, 2.33).*

In general, RP-testing can be applied to those tests whose test statistics follow the Gaussian, the t, the χ^2 and the F distributions, among others.

Furthermore, approximated RP-testing can be applied to the test whose test statistic is approximately Z, or t, or χ^2, or F distributed. For example, tests for comparing proportions and those for comparing time-to-event data (e.g., the log-rank test) own a Z distributed large sample test statistic; tests on Cox's proportional hazards model in survival analysis and tests on contingency tables data (e.g. for comparing more than two proportions) have a χ^2 distributed large sample test statistic.

Some of the tests cited above will be developed in Part II, and SP estimation, including RP-testing, will be developed for them.

2.3   The RP estimate and the p-value

The RP estimate and the p-value are not just indexes for evaluating the outcome of the test, but they can both also be used for defining the statistical test itself. They can therefore be compared. In practice, the lower the p-value, the higher the strength of rejecting H_0, the more "stable" the outcome of the test, the higher the RP estimate.

One might argue that the RP estimate is not useful because it does not add any information to the p-value. This is true: both these indexes are a function of the test statistic, which contains the entire available information. So, not even the p-value adds any information to the test statistic. Consequently, it may be specularly argued that the p-value does not add any information to $\hat{RP}_\alpha$.

Nevertheless, RP estimation provides a different and new perspective to the outcome of the test. First, it recalls that the test is experimental proof of H_1, which can be either successful or not. Second, it reveals the *randomness* of the outcome of the test: measuring the probability to be significant implies that the outcome is a random one.

Moreover, the RP-approach requires the type I error level α to be fixed before the evaluation of the results of the study. This is also the perspective of regulatory agencies, such as the American FDA. Consequently, the RP estimate depends explicitly on α, whereas the p-value does not.

In order to evaluate the test outcome through the p-value, α is usually looked at, and to evaluate the "stability" of the result the difference between the p-value and α is also looked at. As argued in Section 2.1, this difference is often misleading since it tends to overemphasize statistically significant p-values.

In conclusion, since the $\{0, 1\}$ outcome of the tests has a random nature and represents the result of the experiment, in the spirit of the Scientific Method the reproducibility of the outcome *should* be evaluated and, therefore, the RP estimate should be considered as the *rational* index of the stability of the test result.

The p-value (1.9) and the $\hat{RP}_\alpha$ in (2.1) are a function of the test statistic T_n. These functions are shown in Figure 2.3. Note that both functions are monotone and so they can be inverted.

Consequently, these two indexes are linked: in practice the former can be written as a function of the latter, and vice versa. Indeed, from (1.9) and (2.1) we obtain:

$$\text{p-value} = 1 - \Phi(T_n) = 1 - \Phi(\Phi^{-1}(\hat{RP}_\alpha) + z_{1-\alpha})$$

and

$$\hat{RP}_\alpha = \Phi(T_n - z_{1-\alpha}) = \Phi(\Phi^{-1}(1 - \text{p-value}) - z_{1-\alpha})$$

As one can see, $\hat{RP}_\alpha$ increases as the p-value decreases. Moreover, at a given p-value, $\hat{RP}_\alpha$ increases if the type I error increases: $\hat{RP}_\alpha < \hat{RP}_{\alpha'}$ with $\alpha < \alpha'$. This means that given a certain result, the larger the type I error probability is allowed to be, the higher the RP is estimated. These two concepts are well reported in Figure 2.4, where some RP estimates at different α levels are shown as functions of the p-value.

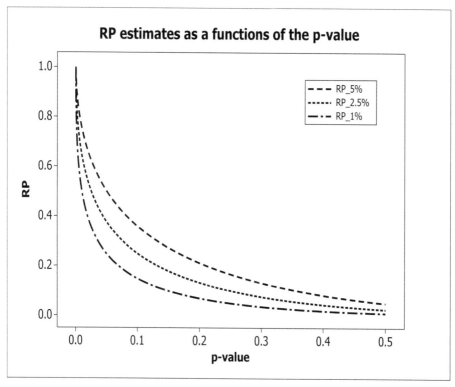

Figure 2.4   *RP estimates with different αs showed as a function of the p-value, for the Z-test.*

As argued through Example 2.1, the distance between the p-value and α is often misleading since it tends to overemphasize statistically significant p-values. A numerical example of these concepts, i.e. the relation between the two indexes and α, is provided below.

■ **EXAMPLE 2.3**

Let us continue Example 2.1. Recall that the test statistic resulted 2.17 and the p-value was 1.5%. *Also, the estimated RP with the type I error set at* 2.5% *was:*

Table 2.1   p-values and pointwise RP estimates for the Z-test with different α levels (i.e. $\hat{RP}_\alpha$), for different values of the Z distributed test statistic.

Test statistic		Type I error level α		
Z	p-value	5%	2.5%	1%
0.842	0.2	21.09%	13.17%	6.88%
1.282	0.1	35.82%	24.88%	14.81%
1.645	0.05	50.00%	37.63%	24.78%
1.751	0.04	54.21%	41.71%	28.24%
1.881	0.03	59.33%	46.84%	32.80%
1.960	0.025*	62.37%	50.00%	35.70%
2.054	0.02	65.87%	53.74%	39.26%
2.326	0.01	75.22%	64.30%	50.00%
2.576	0.005**	82.41%	73.10%	59.85%
2.807	0.0025	87.74%	80.15%	68.46%
3.090	0.001	92.58%	87.08%	77.75%
3.227	0.000625	94.32%	89.75%	81.62%
3.291	0.0005***	95.01%	90.83%	83.25%
3.719	0.0001	98.10%	96.07%	91.81%
4.265	10^{-5}	99.56%	98.94%	97.37%
4.753	10^{-6}	99.91%	99.74%	99.24%
5.199	10^{-7}	99.98%	99.94%	99.80%

$\hat{RP}_{2.5\%} = 58.3\%$. *Increasing α up to 5% we obtained $\hat{RP}_{5\%} = 70.0\%$ (see Table B.1). It is worth noting that although the p-value looks, in this case, quite far from $\alpha = 5\%$, it is estimated that there is a 30% probability of finding a non-significant result in an identical replication of the experiment. When $\alpha = 1\%$, the test is not significant and we find $\hat{RP}_{1\%} = 43.8\%$, which is lower than $1/2$ in accordance with RP-testing equation (2.2).*

Table 2.1 reports p-values and RP estimates for $\alpha = 5\%, 2.5\%$ and 1% for some values of the test statistic. Some asterisks are also reported at some p-values, according to the traditional asterisk scale: (*), (**) and (***) meaning mild, moderate and high statistically significance (see also Section 2.6). First, it should be noted that when the test is significant and the p-value is very close to α (i.e. a bit lower) the estimated RP is approximately 50%. This might by surprising, but this is so. When the p-value moves from α for a quantity which might be considered to be quite a bit, the RP may still be quite low. For example, when $\alpha = 2.5\%$ the p-values of 2% and 1% provide RP estimates of just 53.74% and 64.30%, respectively. For the latter type I error level the outcomes seem to become "stable" for p-values around (and lower than) 0.0005, that is, such that the RP is estimated to be around (and even higher than) 90%.

Note that these RP values are realizations of the *pointwise* RP estimator, which does not take into account the variability of the samples.

2.4 Statistical lower bounds for the RP

Since the variability of RP estimates should be taken into account, we have to equip RP estimation with confidence intervals (Section 1.2). From a conservative perspective, the lowest admissible values are of interest, that are lower bounds of confidence intervals (namely, statistical lower bounds). This conservative approach reflects on the need of one-sided confidence intervals for RP.

In order to perform this conservative estimation, it is necessary to define the percentage γ of the confidence level of the interval. This γ is the probability that the statistical lower bound falls below the unknown RP.

Then, γ-lower bounds for RP can be obtained, and they can be used to evaluate the outcomes of statistical tests and the variability of the latter outcomes.

Referring to the two-sample Z-test, confidence intervals are first computed on δ_t, and then transferred on the RP estimate, which is, in fact, a function of the estimate of δ_t. Our interest in *stability* implies focusing on the lowest admissible values for RP. Then, one-sided confidence intervals for RP can be obtained through one-sided confidence intervals for δ_t. (In the same way, pointwise RP estimates have been obtained in Section 2.1 through pointwise estimates of δ_t, by exploiting the plug-in principle.)

Recall that, from (1.4), a γ-lower bound for δ_t is $d_n^\gamma = d_n - z_\gamma \sqrt{2/n}$. Then, a lower bound for RP (i.e. a conservative estimator for RP) is obtained through the plug-in of d_n^γ in the power function (1.7) and, hence, it results:

$$\hat{RP}_\alpha^\gamma = P_{d_n^\gamma}(T_n^* > z_{1-\alpha} \,|\, T_n) = \Phi(T_n - z_\gamma - z_{1-\alpha}) \tag{2.3}$$

$\hat{RP}_\alpha^\gamma$ is a γ-lower bound for RP (i.e. a γ-conservative estimator). When $\gamma = 50\%$ the so called *median* estimator is obtained. Since $z_{50\%} = 0$, with the Z-test the median estimator coincides with the pointwise estimator, i.e. $\hat{RP}_\alpha^{50\%} = \hat{RP}_\alpha$. This $\hat{RP}_\alpha^\gamma$ is a function of T_n, and so, thanks to (1.9) and (2.3), and in analogy with $\hat{RP}_\alpha$ (as shown in Section 2.3), it can be viewed as a function of the p-value. In Figure 2.5 the values of some conservative estimates for RP, together with the pointwise one, are shown for small p-values. Note that $\hat{RP}_\alpha^{90\%}$ (i.e. the less conservative estimator) begins to be higher than $1/2$ (i.e. the threshold of statistical significance for RP-testing) with p-values around 0.0005.

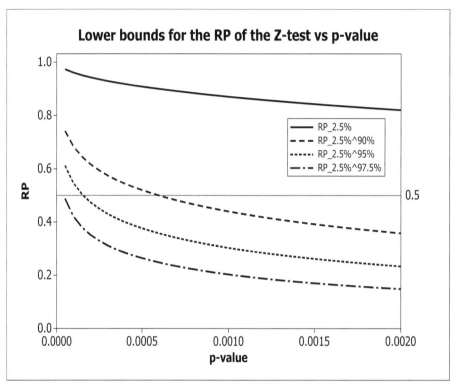

Figure 2.5 *Conservative RP estimates as a function of the p-value, for the Z-test with* $\alpha = 2.5\%$.

■ **EXAMPLE 2.4**

Let us continue Example 2.1, where $d_{85} = 0.333$ and $T_{85} = 2.17$. Since $z_{90\%} = 1.281$, the 90% lower bound for δ_t, i.e. the 90%-conservative estimate, results $0.333 - 1.281 \times \sqrt{2/85} = 0.136$ (use (1.4)). Remember that $\alpha = 2.5\%$ was set and that the pointwise estimated RP resulted $\hat{RP}_{2.5\%} = 58.3\%$. The 90%-conservative estimate of RP is, according to (2.3), $\hat{RP}_{2.5\%}^{90\%} = 14.2\%$ (also Table B.5 can be used, with $T_{85} = 2.17$). The 95% and 97.5% conservative estimates resulted 7.6% (see Table B.6) and 4.0%, respectively.

2.5 The γ-stability criterion for statistical significance

The variability of the test outcomes represents a serious concern. It happens quite frequently that different studies on a certain drug provide inconsistent results. This means that in some studies the results are statistically significant (i.e. the positive effect of the drug is experimentally proved) whereas in some others they are not. Of course, the latter results do not imply that a null effect of the drug is proved, but only that the effect of the drug is not proved.

Stability criteria for statistically significant outcomes are, therefore, very useful. For example, the distance of the p-value from the threshold of statistical significance (i.e. α) is often taken into account. This difference has been ranked into the so-called "asterisk scale" of the p-value (see Section 2.6 for details), which represents the stability criterion traditionally adopted, even in the context of medical statistics.

However, what is *stability*?

Given the $\{0, 1\}$ randomness of the outcomes (i.e. given the Bernoullian nature) of the test, and given that a statistically significant result (i.e. $\{1\}$) represents an experimental proof of effectiveness, stability should be linked to a $\{1\}$ result which has low variability. That is to say that *stability* should be viewed in terms of high reproducibility of the outcome $\{1\}$. This leads directly to the evaluation of stability in terms of RP estimation.

When RP-testing is adopted, the statistical significance is observed if the RP estimate is greater than $1/2$. Then, by considering the variability of RP estimates, statistical lower bounds for RP (i.e. conservative estimates for RP) can be compared with the threshold of statistical significance at $1/2$. Hence, if the lower bound for RP is over $1/2$ the statistical significance can be considered stable.

In this context, γ represents the amount of conservativeness adopted in the lower bound for RP. If the γ-lower bound for RP falls above $1/2$ then the γ-*stability of the statistical significance of the test* is observed. Hence, γ-stability controls the variability of statistically significant outcomes.

Even if in a certain trial a γ-stable outcome is found, the possibility that the null hypothesis is true, and a type I error is committed, actually exists.

In practice, the type I error probabilities together with the probabilities of a stability outcome in the first study and a significant/non-significant one in the second study are about two orders of magnitude smaller than the prefixed α.

The possibility, under the alternative hypothesis, of finding a γ-stable result in the first study and a non-significant one in the second study also exists. The probability of this event results, at maximum, around 5%.

Finally, γ-stability is often applied by adopting $\gamma = 90\%$, and so it becomes 90%-stability.

Formally speaking, being $\hat{RP}_\alpha^\gamma$ the γ-conservative estimator of RP, it follows that from the RP-testing equation 2.2 a γ-conservative result for the statistical significance of the test is:

$$\hat{RP}_\alpha^\gamma > 1/2$$

This result is called γ-*stability of the statistical significance of the test* (De Martini, 2012).

In order to remark on the dependency of this definition on the level α of the test, it might also be said that *the statistical significance of a statistical test is γ-stable with respect to α*.

As a further explanation, consider first that the RP-test (2.2) can be written as a function of the pointwise RP estimator:

$$\psi_\alpha(\hat{RP}_\alpha) = \begin{cases} 1 & \text{if} \quad \hat{RP}_\alpha > 1/2 \\ 0 & \text{if} \quad \hat{RP}_\alpha \leq 1/2 \end{cases} \tag{2.4}$$

Then, accounting for the variability of $\hat{RP}_\alpha$, consider the interval $(\hat{RP}_\alpha^\gamma, 1]$, i.e. the set of "at worst" γ-confident values for RP. Now, applying the RP-test (2.4) to the elements of the latter set, the set of "at worst" γ-confident values for the outcome of the test is obtained. So, if the worst RP estimate is statistically significant (i.e. $\hat{RP}_\alpha^\gamma > 1/2$), then all the "at worst" γ-confident outcomes of the test are statistically significant. In other words, γ-stability is observed when only significant outcomes are γ-confident.

Usually, γ is chosen in accordance with standard levels of confidence, e.g. $\gamma = 90\%, 95\%, 97.5\%$. Also, note that 50%-stability with respect to α turns out to be, simply, the statistical significance at the level α.

Remark 2.1. *γ-stability can be iterated. Through hypothesis testing, the alternative H_1 regarding the effectiveness of the new drug can be experimentally proved. The eventual statistical significance can be viewed as a zero-order stability of the proof. Then, since the test (i.e. the experimental proof) contains randomness, a γ-confidence based proof of the statistical significance is provided by γ-stability. This is the first-order of γ-stability. Even the latter result is subject to random variation and its stability can, therefore, be analyzed. Going further, second-order stability may be evaluated, that is γ'-stability on γ-stability, and so on.*

Iteration is not a new concept in statistics. For example, the well known bootstrap method (that will be applied in Part II to estimate the SP in the nonparametric framework) can be iterated. In particular, iterated bootstrap may be applied to reduce the bias in pointwise estimation or to improve coverage accuracy of asymptotic confidence intervals (Hall and Martin, 1988, Martin, 1990).

◼ **EXAMPLE 2.5**

Let us continue Example 2.4. Considering $\gamma = 90\%$, $\hat{RP}_{2.5\%}^{90\%} = 14.2\% < 1/2$ was obtained, so the test outcome is not 90%-stable with respect to the type I error of 2.5%. If $\alpha = 5\%$ had been set, $\hat{RP}_{5\%}^{90\%} = 22.5\%$ would have been obtained (see Table B.2); so, not even with this (higher) α would the outcome be 90%-stable.

Let us now assume that the sample average of the first population was 0.649, so the estimated effect size was $d_{85} = 0.649 - 0.144 = 0.505$. Then, the test statistic would be $T_{85} = \sqrt{85/2} \times 0.505 = 3.29$ and consequently the test was "highly significant": the p-value, indeed, would be 0.0005 (i.e. *** in the asterisk scale). In this case the RP estimate would be $\hat{RP}_{2.5\%} = 90.8\%$ (see Table B.4), and its 90%-conservative estimate would result $\hat{RP}_{2.5\%}^{90\%} = 51.9\%$ (see Table B.5), which is greater than $1/2$ (i.e. the threshold of significance for RP-testing). So, in this case the statistical significance would be 90%-stable.

2.5.1 γ-stability and type I errors

It is possible to observe a γ-stable outcome (i.e. $\hat{RP}_\alpha^\gamma > 1/2$) even under the null. In this case, considering the outcome significant (and stable), a type I error occurs. The probabilities of finding a γ-stable outcome under the null are, at most, $\alpha_\gamma = P_{\delta_t=0}(\hat{RP}_\alpha^\gamma > 1/2)$, whose values are reported in Table 2.2.

Since pharmaceutical companies often conduct two independent trials, sometimes almost simultaneously, the probability of finding, under H_0, a γ-stable result in the first trial and a non-significant result in the second one with identical settings, resulting in $\alpha_\gamma \times (1-\alpha)$, is also reported. Furthermore, Table 2.2 provides the probabilities, once again under the null, to find a γ-stable result in the first trial and a simple statistical significance in the second one (i.e. $\alpha_\gamma \times \alpha$).

For example, with $\alpha = 2.5\%$, if the null hypothesis is true the probability of finding a 90%-stable result is 0.0594%, finding a 90%-stable result in the first trial and a non-significant result in the second one is 0.0580% and finding a 90%-stable result in the first trial and a simple statistical significance in the second one is 0.0015%.

2.5.2 γ-stability and type II errors

Under H_1 there also exists the possibility of finding a γ-stable result in the first study and a type II error in the second study, i.e. a non-significant outcome. The probability of this inconsistent result can be viewed as a function of RP, i.e. the true power. Through simple algebra it can be shown that the latter probability turns out

Table 2.2   Probabilities of observing γ-stable outcomes under the null hypothesis, for the one-tailed Z-test.

		Type I error level α		
		5%	2.5%	1%
	α_γ	0.1715%	0.0594%	0.0154%
$\gamma = 90\%$	$\alpha_\gamma \times (1 - \alpha)$	0.1672%	0.0580%	0.0150%
	$\alpha_\gamma \times \alpha$	0.0043%	0.0015%	0.0004%
	α_γ	0.0501%	0.0156%	0.0036%
$\gamma = 95\%$	$\alpha_\gamma \times (1 - \alpha)$	0.0489%	0.0152%	0.0035%
	$\alpha_\gamma \times \alpha$	0.0013%	0.0004%	0.0001%
	α_γ	0.0156%	0.0044%	0.0009%
$\gamma = 97.5\%$	$\alpha_\gamma \times (1 - \alpha)$	0.0152%	0.0043%	0.0009%
	$\alpha_\gamma \times \alpha$	0.0004%	0.0001%	$< 0.0001\%$

to be:

$$P(\{\hat{RP}_\alpha^\gamma > 1/2\}_{1st} \text{ and } \{\hat{RP}_\alpha \leq 1/2\}_{2nd}) = (1 - \Phi(z_\gamma - z_{RP})) \times (1 - RP)$$

Note that the above quantity does not depend on α. Moreover, the probability is a concave function of RP, as Figure 2.6 shows. For example, with $\gamma = 90\%$ the probability of finding a γ-stable result in the first study and a type II error in the second one assumes its maximum of 6.8% which corresponds to an RP of 73.9%; with an RP of 90%, 95%, the probability value reduces to 5%, 3.2%, respectively.

2.6   Other stability criteria for statistical significance

Besides γ-stability, some other stability criteria for statistically significant outcomes of the tests exist.

Two of them are based on p-values: one is the traditional asterisk scale; the other (viz. α^2-stability) refers to the overall type I error of two studies (i.e. α^2), in order to reduce the type I error of one study to that of two studies.

Two other criteria are based on RP estimates (the pointwise and the conservative ones, viz. G-stability and S&C-stability, respectively), and they refer to one of the standard thresholds often adopted for the power in sample size determination (see Section 3.1), that is 90%: in practice, the outcome of a trial is considered stable when the probability that a second trial would be significant is estimated (pointwise or conservatively) to be at least 90%.

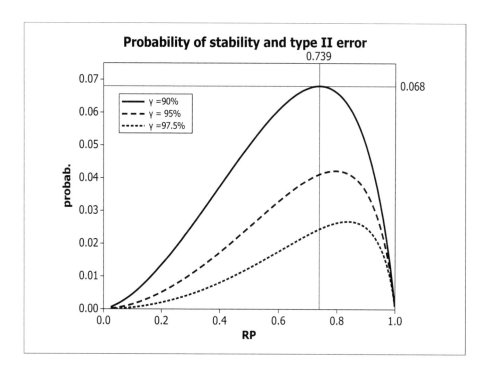

Figure 2.6 *Probability of finding γ-stability in the first trial and a type II error in the second trial, as a function of the RP for the one-tailed Z-test.*

Regulatory agencies, such as the American FDA and the European EMA, usually require more than one statistically significant study (i.e. a minimum of two significant studies) to demonstrate effectiveness of a new treatment.

The main application of stability evaluations in the context of clinical trials is to show *stability* of significant outcomes with one study, in order to avoid other confirmatory studies. (This possibility, i.e. the regulatory position of FDA and EMA, will be explained in-depth in Section 2.8.)

Apart from the asterisk scale, the criteria introduced here are based on concepts that involve a second study. Moreover, none of these criteria are based on the novelty of RP-testing.

Asterisk scale. This is the traditional way for evaluating the degree of statistical significance. It is widely used in many applied fields, and also in bio-medical research. For one-tailed tests, a (*) result means that the test is significant at the level $\alpha = 2.5\%$, that is the usual type I error requested in clinical trial. (**) and (***) require p-values < 0.005 and < 0.0005, respectively, and indicate an increasing degree of statistical significance.

Often, these asterisk ranks are called a mild, a moderate and a high statistically significant outcome, respectively. The asterisk scale is also used for evaluating the stability of clinical trial outcomes and its steps can be, therefore, called a *mild*, a *moderate* and a *high stability*, with respect to $\alpha = 2.5\%$.

p-value lower than α^2. Stemming from the p-value testing (1.10), where the threshold for significance was the type I error level α, since at least two significant studies are requested by regulatory agencies, the p-value is sometimes referred to the overall type I error probability of two trials. This probability is, when the two studies are independent, equal to α^2. When α is 2.5% the overall type I error probability is 0.0625%. If the p-value results lower than α^2 then this outcome is called the α^2-stability.

This approach has been considered by many authors, among these are Hung and O'Neill (2003). Further consideration regarding the design of the single study which refers to this criterion of stability can be found in Darken and Ho (2004) and in Shun et al. (2005).

Standard thresholds for pointwise RP. Goodman (1992) introduced the use of pointwise RP estimators (i.e. $\hat{RP}_\alpha$) for evaluating the outcome of the experiments. Since RP *is* the true power, he compared RP estimates with the standard thresholds for the power adopted when a new study is planned, that are usually around 90%. Several authors have recently encouraged the adoption of a power not lower than 90% (e.g. Wang et al., 2006), and this is also due to the high rate of phase III trials that do not succeed.

Stemming from Goodman's 1992 remarkable paper, other authors (such as Shao and Chow, 2002, Hung and O'Neill, 2003) suggest considering the outcome of a study as stable if the estimate of the probability of finding statistical significance in a second trial is at least 90%. This criterion which considers stable as an outcome providing $\hat{RP}_\alpha > 90\%$ has been formalized as *G-stability with respect to* α, where G stands for Goodman.

Standard thresholds for conservative RP. Shao and Chow (2002) went further than Goodman's pointwise RP estimates and, being aware of the variability of the pointwise estimator $\hat{RP}_\alpha$, suggested the adoption of the conservative estimates given by $\hat{RP}_\alpha^\gamma$ to be compared with the standard power thresholds used in experimental planning.

In particular, in one of the numerical examples they provided, γ was set equal to 97.5% and the 90% power threshold was used. The criterion which considers an outcome stable if it is estimated (with a conservativeness of $\gamma = 97.5\%$) that a second study would be significant with probability at least 90% (i.e. $\hat{RP}_{\alpha}^{97.5\%} > 90\%$) has been formalized as *S&C-stability with respect to* α (where S&C stands for Shao and Chow).

Remark 2.2. *Through simple algebra, it can be shown that γ-stability introduced in the previous Section is, with $\gamma = 90\%$, equivalent to G-stability. In practice:*

$$\hat{RP}_{\alpha}^{90\%} > 1/2 \quad \text{if and only if} \quad \hat{RP}_{\alpha} > 90\%$$

This equivalence is only valid with the Z-test, which has been adopted for introducing these concepts of RP estimation. In other words, this equivalence holds when the test statistic T_n is normally distributed, and it does not when T_n is, for example, distributed as a Student's t or a χ^2.

2.7 Comparing stability criteria

In order to evaluate which relationships exist among stability criteria, a numerical comparison among the latter has been performed, considering different type I error levels, i.e. $\alpha = 5\%, 2.5\%, 1\%$.

Regarding the asterisk scale, when $\alpha = 2.5\%$ the (***) outcome (i.e. high-stability) results close to G-stability, 90%-stability and α^2-stability. However, when α is different from 2.5%, for example, $\alpha = 1\%$ (as it can be when, in the presence of two primary outcomes, α is split into two smaller αs), the asterisk scale loses its meaning. In these situations a new scale should be introduced, but it is not clear which one.

In general, G-stability, 90%-stability and α^2-stability are quite close, especially when $\alpha = 2.5\%$, where 95%-stability is a bit stricter. S&C stability turns out to be very strict, although it takes α into account.

These findings are confirmed even when the distribution of the test statistic is a t or a χ^2.

Table 2.3 reports the p-values and the conservative RP estimates for different values of the test statistic, not just for $\alpha = 2.5\%$, but also for 5% and 1%. The related pointwise RP estimates can be found in Table 2.1.

At first, the asterisk scale was built for a fixed $\alpha = 2.5\%$, and does not depend on potentially different αs. For example, when $\alpha = 1\%$, what is the meaning of the so-called high-stability (***), that is, a p-value lower than 0.05%? The point is that the traditional asterisk scale assumes some significance only when $\alpha = 2.5\%$.

When $\alpha = 2.5\%$, a (***) outcome is close to the α^2-stability and to the G-stability (which coincides with 90%-stability - Remark 2.2). In detail, the (***) is a bit more severe than these two criteria, since its Z outcome (i.e. 3.291) is a bit higher than those needed for the above stabilities, which are 3.242 for G-stability and 3.227 for α^2-stability (the latter value can be found in Table 2.3). Note, therefore, that α^2-stability is the less stringent one in this case.

On the contrary, the S&C-stability needs quite a high Z, even higher than 5.199 (i.e. the highest Z value reported in Table 2.3), for which we have $\hat{RP}_{2.5\%}^{97.5\%} = 89.86\%$. Regarding 95%- and 97.5%-stability, they are more severe than the first three criteria discussed and, of course, less severe than the S&C-stability. With this α of 2.5%, 95% and 97.5% stabilities occur with $Z = 3.605$ and $Z = 3.920$, respectively.

With a different α the ordering of stabilities changes. With $\alpha = 1\%$ the following order results: high- (i.e. ***), G- (i.e. 90%-), α^2-, 95%-, 97.5%- and S&C-stability, which are obtained with Z equal to 3.608, 3.719, 3.972, 4.287 and 5.568, respectively. With $\alpha = 5\%$ the stability order is α^2-, G- (i.e. 90%-), 95%-, high- (***), 97.5%- and S&C-stability.

In all situations the S&C-stability requires very small p-values: around 10^{-6}, 10^{-7}, 10^{-8} with $\alpha = 5\%, 2.5\%, 1\%$, respectively. This very strict criterion is fulfilled in extreme situations.

These considerations are valid also when the distribution of the test statistic T_n is a t or a χ^2 (see De Martini, 2012). Conservative RP estimates for t distributions will be shown in Chapter 6, and those for the χ^2 ones in Chapter 8. How to compute these estimates will also be explained.

2.8   Regulatory agencies and the single study

In order to assess the quantity of evidence necessary to support effectiveness of a certain treatment, regulatory agencies (viz. the U.S. FDA, the European EMA) usually ask for at least two adequate and well controlled studies. Nevertheless, in some circumstances this two-study requirement is amended.

The FDA Modernization Act of 1997 states that data from one adequate and well-controlled clinical investigation and confirmatory evidence may be sufficient to establish effectiveness. The possibility introduced by this amendment is clearly motivated in the FDA Guidance for Industry of 1998, where many useful examples for explaining the position of this agency are also provided.

Concentration of the document is on:

- a) situations in which a single adequate and well-controlled study of a specific new use can be supported by information from other related adequate and well-controlled studies, such as studies in other phases of a disease, in closely related diseases, of other conditions of use (different dose, duration of use, regimen), of different dosage forms, or of different endpoints;

Table 2.3   p-values and γ-conservative RP estimates for the one-tailed Z-test with different α levels (i.e. $\hat{RP}_\alpha^\gamma$), for different values of the Z distributed test statistic. (When $\alpha = 1\%$, the α^2 line for evaluating α^2-stability coincides with the p-value 0.0001.)

	Z	p-value	$\hat{RP}_\alpha^{90\%}$	$\hat{RP}_\alpha^{95\%}$	$\hat{RP}_\alpha^{97.5\%}$
$\alpha = 5\%$	1.960	0.025 (*)	16.69%	9.18%	5.00%
	2.576	0.005 (**)	36.30%	23.77%	15.17%
	2.807	$0.0025 = \alpha^2$	45.25%	31.47%	21.25%
	3.291	0.0005 (***)	64.21%	50.03%	37.67%
	3.719	0.0001	78.60%	66.62%	54.55%
	4.753	10^{-6}	96.62%	92.84%	87.46%
	5.199	10^{-7}	98.85%	97.19%	94.46%
$\alpha = 2.5\%$	1.960	0.025 (*)	10.00%	5.00%	2.50%
	2.576	0.005 (**)	25.28%	15.20%	8.94%
	3.227	$0.000625 = \alpha^2$	49.43%	35.29%	24.42%
	3.291	0.0005 (***)	51.96%	37.67%	26.45%
	3.719	0.0001	68.35%	54.55%	42.04%
	4.753	10^{-6}	93.47%	87.46%	79.77%
	5.199	10^{-7}	97.49%	94.46%	89.86%
$\alpha = 1\%$	1.960	0.025 (*)	4.97%	2.22%	1.00%
	2.576	0.005 (**)	15.10%	8.15%	4.36%
	3.291	0.0005 (***)	37.55%	24.80%	15.97%
	3.719	$0.0001 = \alpha^2$	54.42%	40.04%	28.53%
	4.753	10^{-6}	87.40%	78.30%	67.98%
	5.199	10^{-7}	94.42%	89.03%	81.94%

- b) situations in which a single multicenter study, without supporting information from other adequate and well-controlled studies, may provide evidence that a use is effective.

The two situations described above are different, as are the statistical results required; in the former case no particular emphasis is placed on statistical results that should be significant, while in the latter one, besides some important considerations about the design of the study, the population and the consistency about its subsets, strong statistical results are needed. In other words, findings which are statistically very persuasive are required from the single study (SS). The position of EMA is analogous, even if it is claimed and explained more concisely (see EMEA ICH-09 of 1998, and EMEA-CPMP of 2001).

The stability criteria presented in this Chapter, which has been numerically compared in Section 2.7, represent the statistical techniques for assessing if findings are statistically very persuasive, i.e. for assessing quantity of evidence with an SS.

Regulatory guidelines inherent to very persuasive findings do not mention a virtual second study to which the results of an SS should refer. In particular, a second study is not mentioned either concerning the type I error (eventually of the overall first and second study), or concerning the estimated probability of a second positive outcome.

It follows that although α^2-stability (based on the overall type I error), G-stability and S&C-stability (based on the overtaking of the threshold of 90% by the estimated RP) might be of some interest as a stability criteria, they do not directly reflect the agencies' views. A new element with respect to regulatory guidelines has been introduced for defining these stability criteria, and that is the second potential trial.

The asterisk scale focuses on the strength of the outcome of an SS, and so it conforms to the agencies' views. Nevertheless, admitting that high-stability (i.e. (***)) would be considered a very persuasive finding with a one-tailed test with $\alpha = 2.5\%$, it is not clear how the asterisk scale should be modified with different type I errors.

The γ-stability criterion, which is achieved when all γ-confident outcomes of the test are statistically significant, seems to be more appropriate to evaluate whether or not findings of an SS are very persuasive (provided that γ is set high). It reflects the positions of agencies requiring strong results of an SS more closely than other approaches.

Although the RP perspective is also the basis for this stability criterion, it might recall the eventual results of a second study, the γ-stability criterion consists of a reliability measure of the outcome of the test of only the SS.

2.9 The RP for two-tailed tests

In this Section the statistical tools related to RP estimation introduced in this Chapter will be extended to the two-tailed setting.

2.9.1 RP estimation for two-tailed tests

The probability to prove that one of the drugs is more effective than the other one, avoiding the type III error, is the two-tailed SP (see Section 1.7.2).

Assuming that two samples are available from the two populations in study, in analogy with the one-tailed situation, the SP of a trial based on samples of sizes equal to those available can be viewed as the RP of the ongoing trial. This can be estimated, and its estimates will be denoted by $\hat{RP}_{2;\alpha}$.

The estimates of the *two-tailed RP* turn out to be equal to those of the one-tailed one when the absolute value of the observed effect size is considered and the type I error probability for the one-tailed RP is the halved type I error probability of the two-tailed (i.e. $\alpha/2$).

In analogy with the one-tailed setting, *the RP for the two-tailed test is the true value of the good power, that is the "good power function" evaluated at δ_t.*

Let us assume that two samples of size n are drawn up and that SP_2 in (1.15) is considered. The RP estimator is assumed to be the estimator of the SP. Therefore, the probability on the tail of the Z-distribution where T_n falls is estimated. The pointwise estimator of RP for the two-tailed test is:

$$\hat{RP}_{2;\alpha} = \begin{cases} P_{d_n}(T_n^* > z_{1-\alpha/2} \mid T_n) & \text{if} \quad T_n > 0 \\ P_{d_n}(T_n^* < z_{\alpha/2} \mid T_n) & \text{if} \quad T_n < 0 \end{cases}$$

Since $T_n = d_n \sqrt{n/2}$, the previous equation becomes:

$$\hat{RP}_{2;\alpha} = P_{|d_n|}(T_n^* > z_{1-\alpha/2} \mid T_n) \tag{2.5}$$

In practice, from (2.5) and (2.1) the RP for the two-tailed setting is equal to the one-tailed RP with halved type I error probability, and where it is considered the absolute value of observed effect size (or of the test statistic):

$$\hat{RP}_{2;\alpha} = \Phi(|T_n| - z_{1-\alpha/2}) = \hat{RP}_{\alpha/2} \tag{2.6}$$

2.9.2 Two-tailed RP-testing and relationship with the p-value

RP-testing can even be performed in the two-tailed setting by referring to the point estimate $\hat{RP}_{2;\alpha}$ whose threshold for statistical significance is still $1/2$.

The interpretation of RP-testing in Section 2.2 is, therefore, still valid: *the null hypothesis H_0 is rejected when it is estimated that there is a higher probability to reject it than to accept it.*

In this two-tailed framework the RP estimate and the p-value are still linked, and the former can be viewed as a function of the latter, and vice versa. It should also be noted that neither of these indexes contain the same information of the test statistic, whose sign information (i.e. $+/-$) is lost.

Formally speaking, thanks to the equation (2.6) the threshold for RP-testing is still $1/2$, even in this two-tailed context:

$$\psi_\alpha(T_n) = \begin{cases} 1 & \text{if} \quad \hat{RP}_{2;\alpha} > 1/2 \\ 0 & \text{if} \quad \hat{RP}_{2;\alpha} \leq 1/2 \end{cases} \tag{2.7}$$

As in the one-tailed setting, $\hat{RP}_{2;\alpha}$ and the p-value are linked. Their relationships, thanks to (1.16) and (2.6), modify as follows:

$$\hat{RP}_{2;\alpha} = \Phi(|T_n| - z_{1-\alpha/2}) = \Phi(\Phi^{-1}(1 - \text{p-value}/2) - z_{1-\alpha/2})$$

and

$$\text{p-value} = 2(1 - \Phi(|T_n|)) = 2(1 - \Phi(\Phi^{-1}(\hat{RP}_{2;\alpha}) + z_{1-\alpha/2}))$$

2.9.3 Two-tailed stability criteria

In the two-tailed setting, the criteria for stability evaluations change technically, not conceptually.

The asterisk scale indicates significant results at 5%, 1% and 0.1%, with (*), (**) and (***), respectively. G-stability considers the pointwise estimate of the two-tailed RP (i.e. $\hat{RP}_{2;\alpha}$) to be compared with the threshold of 90%. S&C-stability considers the 97.5% conservative estimate of the two-tailed RP (namely $\hat{RP}_{2;\alpha}^{97.5\%}$) to be compared with 90%. γ-stability looks at the γ-conservative estimate of the two-tailed RP (namely $\hat{RP}_{2;\alpha}^{\gamma}$) with respect to $1/2$, being γ usually equal to 90%, 95% and 97.5%.

The α^2-stability criterion changes as follows: two statistically significant results are needed, but they must both be on the same side. In other words, the p-value should be related to the type I error made if two subsequent significant results are observed, both in favor of the same drug.

Concerning conservative RP estimation, in accordance with the relation between the one- and two-tailed pointwise RP estimators in (2.6), when $T_n > 0$ the γ-conservative estimator (namely $\hat{RP}_{2;\alpha}^{\gamma}$) results equal to $\hat{RP}_{\alpha/2}^{\gamma}$, which can be obtained through (2.3). In general: $\hat{RP}_{2;\alpha}^{\gamma} = P_{|d_n|^{\gamma}}(T_n^* > z_{1-\alpha/2} | T_n)$, where $|d_n|^{\gamma} = |d_n| - z_{\gamma}\sqrt{2/n}$. This results in $\hat{RP}_{2;\alpha}^{\gamma} = \Phi(|T_n| - z_{\gamma} - z_{1-\alpha/2})$, which recalls (2.3).

The "p-value lower than α^2" rule needs the (two-tailed) p-value to be lower than α twice, both on the same tail. This is reflected by the need of the p-value to be lower than $(\alpha/2)^2 \times 2$: in fact, the threshold for the one-tailed p-value (i.e. $\alpha/2$) is squared (because of the two independent significance needed) and multiplied by 2 (which stands for the number of tails). Then, the threshold of α^2-stability for the two-tailed p-value results $\alpha^2/2$ (see, for example, Darken and Ho 2004).

In Table 2.4 some absolute values of the test statistic T_n are reported, together with their respective values of the two-tailed p-value, of the two-tailed pointwise and conservative RP estimates, with $\gamma = 90\%$, 95% and 97.5%. The values of the test statistic which fulfill the different stability criteria with $\alpha = 5\%$ are equal to those that provided stability in the one-tailed setting with $\alpha = 2.5\%$. Consequently, the discussion about the comparison of stability results in Section 2.7 remains valid.

2.10   Discussing Situation I in Section I.4.1

At this point, the statistical tools needed for answering the questions in Situation I in I.4.1 are disposed of. The test was two-tailed with $\alpha = 5\%$, and its outcome (based on a certain difference between sample means, d_n) resulted significant with a two-tailed p-value of 3%. Consequently, the absolute value of T_n was 2.17, which provided a one-tailed p-value of 1.5%. This implies that the pointwise estimate of RP is $\hat{RP}_{2;5\%} = \hat{RP}_{2.5\%} = 58.32\%$ (use Table B.4). Type III error is therefore estimated to be 0.0018%.

If the observed effect size d_n corresponds to the true one, then the probability to reproduce such an outcome is just 58.32%. Actually, this is the *estimated* reproducibility probability. So, this positive outcome of the test is *estimated* to be quite a fortunate one. Consequently, if the second pivotal trial has to be planned, a suggestion would be to increase the sample size with respect to that adopted in the first trial (i.e. n). Of course, the information provided by this trial can be used to decide how to increase n (as we will show in the next Chapter).

Now, assume again (as in Section I.4.1) that the observed p-value is 1%, that is a two-asterisk outcome (i.e. (**)). This implies an absolute value of T_n of 2.576 and a

Table 2.4   p-values, pointwise and γ-conservative RP estimates for the two-tailed Z-test with $\alpha = 5\%$, for different values of $|Z|$, i.e. the absolute value of the test statistic.

$|Z|$	p-value	$\hat{RP}_{2;5\%}$	$\hat{RP}_{2;5\%}^{90\%}$	$\hat{RP}_{2;5\%}^{95\%}$	$\hat{RP}_{2;5\%}^{97.5\%}$
0.842	0.4	13.17%	-	-	-
1.282	0.2	24.88%	-	-	-
1.645	0.1	37.63%	-	-	-
1.751	0.08	41.71%	-	-	-
1.881	0.06	46.84%	-	-	-
1.960	0.05 (*)	50.00%	10.00%	5.00%	2.50%
2.576	0.01 (**)	73.10%	25.28%	15.20%	8.94%
3.227	$0.00125(\alpha^2/2)$	89.75%	49.43%	35.29%	24.42%
3.291	0.001 (***)	90.83%	51.96%	37.67%	26.45%
3.719	0.0002	96.07%	68.35%	54.55%	42.04%
4.753	2×10^{-6}	99.74%	93.47%	87.46%	79.77%
5.199	2×10^{-7}	99.94%	97.49%	94.46%	89.86%

pointwise estimate of the RP of $\hat{RP}_{2;5\%} = 73.10\%$ (Table 2.4, or B.4). Although the p-value seems quite far from the threshold of significance of 5%, the RP is estimated to be not high enough to avoid the second pivotal trial. Not one of the stability criteria compared in Section 2.7 was fulfilled. Instead, an observed outcome for T_n around 3.3, and even better if around 3.6 (i.e. two-tailed p-values from 0.1% to 0.02% - see Table 2.4) would show, in accordance with many stability criteria, enough reproducibility to ask regulatory agencies to avoid the second confirmatory trial. These concepts and numbers are illustrated in Figure 2.7.

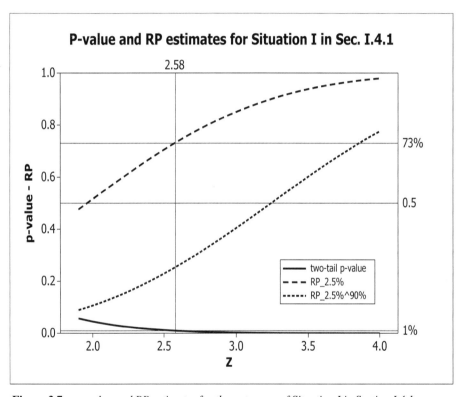

Figure 2.7   *p-value and RP estimates for the outcomes of Situation I in Section I.4.1.*

CHAPTER 3

SAMPLE SIZE ESTIMATION

The planning of an experiment is a crucial point in research, and also in clinical trials development.

A researcher might have the right intuition, but he can only prove it through good experimental planning. Analogously, in clinical trials, a new effective drug can be experimentally proved to be useful through an adequate and well developed scientific protocol.

As shown in the Introduction, it is a fact that approximately 40% of phase III trials fail. This is due to many reasons, as explained in Sections I.2 and I.3, and in some cases to errors in the experimental plan. In particular, wrong assumptions on the effect size can be postulated, which imply a too small sample size and a consequent too low probability of success. Moreover, some phase III trials regarding effective and useful drugs are not launched because phase II data did not show significant results just thanks to bad chance.

Here, focus is placed on one point of the experimental planning of the phase III trial, and that is the computation of the sample size.

Success Probability Estimation with Applications to Clinical Trials, First Edition.
By Daniele De Martini Copyright © 2013 John Wiley & Sons, Inc.

It is a common habit for the information collected during previous phases of the research to be used for planning the following phases (see Guidance for Industry, ICH-E9, 1998). In this context, phase II results and data are used for planning phase III trials.

First, phase III is run only when phase II results are, in some sense, "good enough". Rationalizing this concept, some launch criteria for phase III based on phase II data emerge.

Then, also the sample size of phase III is based on phase II data. Rationalizing this concept, the estimation of phase III sample size, through the estimation of the effect size, on the basis of phase II data becomes evident.

Moreover, the variability of phase II data is very seldom taken into account during these two steps. To consider the variability of phase II data for planning phase III studies in order to control the probability of success leads to *Conservative Sample Size Estimation* (CSSE) strategies.

In this Chapter the classical sample size determination is first recalled. Then, success probability (SP) estimation for adapting/estimating the sample size is presented. Hence, some practical tools are introduced: some launch criteria for phase III; the variability of sample size estimates; the averaged SP of phase III only, once it has been launched (Average Power); the averaged SP of phases II and III considered jointly (Overall Power). Some frequentist CSSE strategies are then presented, giving rise to the optimal CSSE strategy. Some Bayesian CSSE strategies are also presented and a comparison of the performances of all these strategies is provided. Finally, the application of CSSE strategies to the introductive Situations I and II of Section I.4.2 is shown.

The one-tailed setting is adopted for presenting concepts and for showing examples and results, and the balanced sampling is assumed. Generalization in terms of unbalanced sampling is straightforward. Sample size estimation for the two-tailed setting will be shown at the end of the Chapter.

3.1   The classical paradigm of sample size determination

In order to adequately plan a controlled clinical trial, the sample size should be carefully determined since it is related to the probability of success of the experiment, along with consequent ethical and practical implications.

In particular, a certain effect size δ_a (where "a" stands for "assumed") is considered the true one. Sometimes this assumption is made on the basis of available information, such as pilot data.

Setting the type I error probability (α) allowed by the statistical test is also necessary for sample size determination. Often α is 2.5% (5%) in the one-tailed (two-tailed) setting.

Moreover, the desired probability of success of the experiment (i.e. the probability of finding a significant result if the assumed effect size δ_a is actually equal to the true one - δ_t) is set. This quantity is, of course, quite high (usually 80% or 90%), it is denoted by $1 - \beta$ for simplicity and it is sometimes called "power to detect δ_a". Often $1 - \beta$ is simply called the "power".

On the basis of δ_a, α and $1 - \beta$, the sample size is computed: this is *sample size determination*, and the resulting sample size is here named M_a, since it depends on δ_a.

Different sample sizes provide different SPs. If δ_a is equal to the true effect size δ_t, then the SP given by M_a is $1 - \beta$. Since the latter situation is the ideal one, the *ideal* sample size providing an SP of $1 - \beta$ is denoted by M_I.

Regarding the practical aspect of sample size determination, what if δ_a is different from δ_t, which, remember, is unknown?

On one hand, in case the assumed δ_a is lower than δ_t then M_a is higher than M_I. Consequently, SP is higher than $1 - \beta$ (and that may be fine), but many more patients would be recruited, with an increase in the length of time and cost of the trial.

On the other hand, and this is the main concern, when $\delta_a > \delta_t$ (i.e. overly optimistic assumptions have been made) the SP provided by M_a does not achieve $1 - \beta$, and it can result quite a bit lower. In fact, small deviations of δ_a from δ_t can affect the SP substantially.

To determine the sample size for the statistical test (1.6), separate assumptions can be made for the two population means involved in the effect size. Assuming that the latter are μ_{1a} and μ_{2a}, respectively, then $\delta_a = (\mu_{1a} - \mu_{2a})/\sigma$. Alternatively, one can directly postulate a value for δ_a. To ease notations $\sigma = 1$ is considered, in accordance with previous Chapters.

The determined sample size M_a is the minimum sample size for which the power function (1.7), computed at the assumed δ_a, overcomes the probability of success that has been set (i.e the power value $1 - \beta$). Hence:

$$M_a = \min\{m \quad \text{such that} \quad \pi(\alpha, m, \delta_a) > 1 - \beta\}$$

From (1.7), $\pi(\alpha, m, \delta_a) = \Phi(\delta_a \sqrt{m/2} - z_{1-\alpha})$, and so:

$$M_a = \min\{m \quad \text{such that} \quad \Phi(\delta_a \sqrt{m/2} - z_{1-\alpha}) > 1 - \beta\}$$

which, through Φ^{-1} applied to both terms of the inequality above and simple algebra, gives:

$$M_a = \min\{m \quad \text{such that} \quad m > 2((z_{1-\alpha} + z_{1-\beta})/\delta_a)^2\}$$

Being the sample size an integer greater than 1, the formula assumes the well known shape:

$$M_a = \lfloor 2(z_{1-\alpha} + z_{1-\beta})^2/(\delta_a)^2 \rfloor + 1$$

where $\lfloor x \rfloor$ is the integer part of x.

Now, consider the SP in (1.11). At first, in order to emphasize that SP is a function of the sample size, it will be denoted by $SP(m)$. Hence, it should be remarked that M_a does not provide a probability of success of $1 - \beta$, unless δ_a is set equal to the true effect size δ_t. Indeed, with M_a data per group the SP is $SP(M_a) = \pi(\alpha, M_a, \delta_t)$, which achieves $1 - \beta$ only when $\delta_a \geq \delta_t$.

On the contrary, there actually exists a sample size providing an SP of $1 - \beta$: it is called here the *ideal* sample size and is denoted by M_I, where I stands for *ideal*. The latter sample size is defined as follows:

$$M_I = \min\{m \text{ such that } SP(m) > 1-\beta\} = \min\{m \text{ such that } \pi(\alpha, m, \delta_t) > 1-\beta\}$$

giving:

$$M_I = \lfloor 2(z_{1-\alpha} + z_{1-\beta})^2/(\delta_t)^2 \rfloor + 1 \tag{3.1}$$

It is easy to see that $M_a = M_I$ when δ_a is set equal to δ_t.

■ EXAMPLE 3.1

Let us set $\alpha = 2.5\%$ and $1 - \beta = 90\%$. Assuming $\delta_a = 0.5$, the determined sample size M_a resulted equal to 85 (see also Figure 1.5). If $\delta_t = 0.6$, then $M_a = 85$ giving a good SP of $\pi(2.5\%, 85, 0.6) = 97.5\%$, but M_a is also 44% larger than the ideal sample size, which in this case is $M_I = 59$.

Whereas, if δ_t is 0.4, then $M_I = 132$ and, principally, with 85 data per group the actual SP is $SP(85) = \pi(2.5\%, 85, 0.4) = 74.1\%$ only. If $\delta_t = 0.35$ then $M_I = 172$, and with $M_a = 85$ an even worst SP of $\pi(2.5\%, 85, 0.35) = 62.6\%$ is obtained! The values of $SP(m)$ that gave these results are drawn in Figure 3.1.

As a further example, assuming $\delta_a = 0.25$ the M_a resulted equal to 337. If δ_t is 0.2, then $M_I = 526$ and 337 data per group provide an SP of 73.8%. If $\delta_t = 0.15$, then $M_I = 934$, and with $M_a = 337$, $SP(337)$ is equal to, just, 49.5%.

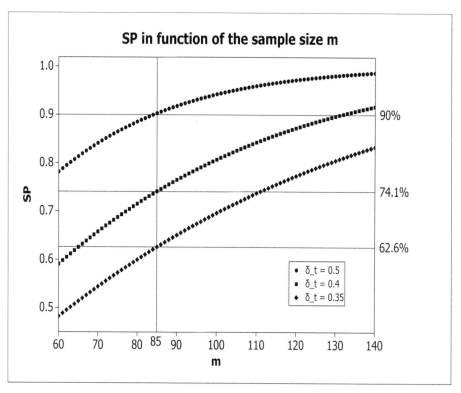

Figure 3.1   *SP in function of the sample size m (viz. $SP(m)$), with $\alpha = 2.5\%$ and $1 - \beta = 90\%$, and with $\delta_t = 0.5, 0.4, 0.35$.*

3.2   SP estimation for adapting the sample size

When some information is available, it can be used to compute a sample size as close as possible to M_I, and so obtain an SP as close as possible to the prefixed power $1 - \beta$.

In practice, when some pilot samples are available (for example, from a phase II) the sample size M_I (for example, for the subsequent phase III) can be adapted on the basis of the estimated SP.

In detail, the SP is estimated at different values of the sample size in order to determine a sample size value as close as possible to M_I. This practice is sometimes called *sample size adaptation by design*, in the sense of adapting the phase II information for planning phase III trials. From a rigorous statistical perspective, in statistical language this is *sample size estimation* (SSE).

For example, the point estimate of the effect size (viz. d_n) can be plugged into the formula of the SP that is used to determine the sample size, obtaining the *pointwise* estimate of the sample size.

Of course, SSE is a consistent technique when the effect size of the population of phase II is equal to that of the phase III population. A sufficient condition is that both studies are performed on the same patient population. This condition is usually fulfilled when the sample size for the second confirmatory phase III trial is estimated on the basis of the data of the first pivotal trial.

Remember that SP is unknown, being dependent on the unknown δ_t. When two samples of size n are available, for example, from a pilot study, SP can be estimated in order to then estimate the ideal sample size for the trial that has to be planned. In order to make reading easier, it is assumed here that the pilot samples come from a phase II study, whereas the trial that is being planned is a phase III one.

Now, let us denote by $\hat{SP}_n^{\bullet}(m)$ a generic estimator of $SP(m)$ (i.e. the SP of a phase III trial with m data per group). Note that the subscript n indicates that $\hat{SP}_n^{\bullet}(m)$ is based on two phase II samples of size n. Then, the generic estimator of the ideal sample size M_I in (3.1) is, therefore:

$$M_n^{\bullet} = \min\{m \quad \text{such that} \quad \hat{SP}_n^{\bullet}(m) > 1 - \beta\} \tag{3.2}$$

This is *sample size estimation*, and it is also called *sample size adaptation by design* by Wang et al. (2006), see also Hung et al. (2006). If $\hat{SP}_n^{\bullet}(m)$ is consistent, then also $M_n^{\bullet}$ is, meaning that its precision in estimating M_I improves as n increases.

Many techniques for estimating SP are available, in the frequentist as well as in the Bayesian framework, and these will be shown later. For example, in the frequentist framework a generic estimator of δ_t (i.e. $d_n^{\bullet}$) can be plugged into the SP equation (1.11), obtaining:

$$\hat{SP}_n^{\bullet}(m) = \pi(\alpha, m, d_n^{\bullet}) \tag{3.3}$$

This is identical to the general SP estimation in (1.12) (only the notation changed). It is remarkable that the definition of the SP estimator based on the plug-in of $d_n^{\bullet}$ is very intuitive and it is often used in practice, as will be shown later. Through (3.2), the latter SP equation gives:

$$M_n^{\bullet} = \lfloor 2(z_{1-\alpha} + z_{1-\beta})^2/(d_n^{\bullet})^2 \rfloor + 1 \tag{3.4}$$

As a particular case of equation (3.4), consider the pointwise estimator of the effect size (i.e. $d_n^{\bullet} = d_n = \bar{X}_{1,n} - \bar{X}_{2,n}$) to be plugged in. Then, the above sample size estimator becomes:

$$M_n = \lfloor 2(z_{1-\alpha} + z_{1-\beta})^2 / (d_n)^2 \rfloor + 1 \qquad (3.5)$$

This is the most intuitive estimator, and it is named the *pointwise sample size estimator*. This approach has been often adopted in the literature, see, for example, Rosner (2005, Chapter 8).

■ EXAMPLE 3.2

Rejoining Situation II in Section I.4.2. During a phase II trial, two samples of size $n = 59$ were collected and they provided an observed effect size (i.e. d_{59}) of 0.48. The type I error for phase III was $\alpha = 2.5\%$ and the power was $1 - \beta = 90\%$. The sample size estimated by the pointwise estimator is, therefore, $M_{59} = \lfloor 2(1.96 + 1.28)^2 / (0.48)^2 \rfloor + 1 = 92$ data per group.

3.3 Launching the trial in practice

Not all the clinical trials of phase II proceed into phase III. The launch of the phase III trial might be subordinate to phase II results, for example, to an eventual statistical significance, or to an observed effect size of some clinical relevance. More prosaically, it happens that phase III is only launched if the estimated costs can be covered by the budget of the trial (i.e. if the estimated sample size is lower than the maximum admitted sample size $M_{\max}$).

The probability to launch phase III, given that the new drug is effective (i.e. $\delta_t > 0$), can be viewed as the SP of phase II.

There are, in practice, some different criteria for launching phase III. Three of them are presented and it is shown that they are mathematically equivalent, in the sense that the parameters of their respective launching rules can be set in order to make them equivalent.

When a technique for SSE meets a launching rule, which subordinates the eventual estimation of the sample size, an SSE *strategy* arises.

Let us denote the random event of the phase III launch by $\mathcal{L}$. The probability to launch when $\delta_t > 0$ is the SP of phase II: $SP_{II} = P_{\delta_t}(\mathcal{L})$.

The statistical significance launch criterion. Phase III is launched if phase II resulted statistically significant, with respect to an appropriate phase II type I error probability, α_{II}. It would be reasonable to allow for values of α_{II} higher than the αs of phase III (e.g. $\alpha_{II} = 10\% - 20\%$). This is due to the fact that at this stage of the research it may be important to avoid the possibility of losing valid new treatments.

Through this approach we have:

$$\mathcal{L} \quad \text{iff} \quad T_n > z_{1-\alpha_{II}}$$

where, we recall, $T_n = d_n \sqrt{n/2}$.

The clinical relevance launch criterion. Phase III is launched if the estimated effect size is larger than an effect size of a certain clinical relevance, namely δ_{0L}. The latter quantity can, in practice, vary over quite a large range, because it depends on clinical considerations regarding the disease that is being studied. Then:

$$\mathcal{L} \quad \text{iff} \quad d_n^\bullet > \delta_{0L}$$

The maximum sample size launch criterion. Assume, first, that there exists the maximum admitted sample size $M_{\max}$. This sample size threshold might depend, for example, on a constraint originated by the trial budget, or by the potentiality of patient recruitment. Then, phase III is launched if the estimated sample size is lower than $M_{\max}$. In formulas:

$$\mathcal{L} \quad \text{iff} \quad M_n^\bullet \leq M_{\max}$$

3.3.1   Equivalence of launching criteria

Assume $d_n^\bullet$ to be an increasing function (say h) of the observed effect size d_n, that is $d_n^\bullet = h(d_n)$, where $h(x_1) < h(x_2)$ with $x_1 < x_2$. Hence, the launching criteria can be set in order to be mathematically equivalent.

Now, supposing that α_{II} is given:

$$T_n > z_{1-\alpha_{II}} \quad \text{iff} \quad d_n > z_{1-\alpha_{II}}\sqrt{2/n} \quad \text{iff} \quad h(d_n) = d_n^\bullet > h(z_{1-\alpha_{II}}\sqrt{2/n})$$

That is, the clinical relevance criterion is equivalent to the statistical significance one, when:

$$\delta_{0L} = h(z_{1-\alpha_{II}}\sqrt{2/n}) \tag{3.6}$$

Specularly, supposing that δ_{0L} is given, the statistical significance criterion is equivalent to the second one when $\alpha_{II} = 1 - \Phi(\sqrt{n/2}\,h^{-1}(\delta_{0L}))$.

When the SP estimator is obtained by plugging $d_n^\bullet$ into the power function, so that $\hat{SP}_n^\bullet(m) = \pi(\alpha, m, d_n^\bullet)$, it can be shown that the maximum sample size criterion is equivalent to the clinical relevance one. Supposing $M_{\max}$ given, from (3.4) we have:

$$M_n^\bullet \leq M_{\max} \quad \text{iff} \quad \left\lfloor \frac{2(z_{1-\alpha} + z_{1-\beta})^2}{(d_n^\bullet)^2} \right\rfloor + 1 \leq M_{\max}$$

$$\text{iff} \quad \frac{2(z_{1-\alpha} + z_{1-\beta})^2}{(d_n^\bullet)^2} < M_{\max}$$

$$\text{iff} \quad d_n^{\bullet} > \sqrt{2/M_{\max}}(z_{1-\alpha} + z_{1-\beta}) \quad \text{iff} \quad d_n > h^{-1}(\sqrt{2/M_{\max}}(z_{1-\alpha} + z_{1-\beta}))$$

That is: the clinical relevance criterion is equivalent to the maximum sample size one when $\delta_{0L} = h^{-1}(\sqrt{2/M_{\max}}(z_{1-\alpha} + z_{1-\beta}))$. Specularly, supposing that δ_{0L} is given, the third criterion is equivalent to the second one when:

$$M_{\max} = \lfloor 2(z_{1-\alpha} + z_{1-\beta})^2/(d_{0L})^2 \rfloor + 1 \tag{3.7}$$

3.3.2 Numerical comparison of launching criteria

At first, note that the condition $d_n^{\bullet} = h(d_n)$ is fulfilled for all the conservative estimators of δ_t of the form $d_n^{\gamma} = d_n - z_{\gamma}\sqrt{2/n}$. These are, remember, the lower bounds of one-directional confidence intervals of δ_t (see (1.4) in Section 1.2).

In Table 3.1 some numerical relationships among launching criteria are reported. Given a sample size n and an effect size threshold δ_{0L}, the phase II type I error level α_{II} is computed according to (3.6), with $h(d_n) = d_n^{\gamma}$, for $\gamma = 50\%, 75\%, 84.1\%$ - the adoption of the latter two values of γ will be explained later. $M_{\max}$ is also given, depending on δ_{0L} only (see (3.7)). Note that α_{II} is quite low in correspondence of high launch threshold and amount of conservativeness (i.e. $\delta_{0L} \geq 0.2$ and $\gamma \geq 75\%$).

Table 3.1 Numerical relationships among launching criteria, with $\alpha = 2.5\%, 1 - \beta = 90\%$.

n	δ_{0L}	$M_{\max}$	phase II type I error - α_{II}		
			$d_n^{\bullet} = d_n$	$d_n^{\bullet} = d_n^{75\%}$	$d_n^{\bullet} = d_n^{84.1\%}$
	0.1	2102	29.19%	11.08%	6.10%
	0.15	934	20.57%	6.73%	3.44%
60	0.2	526	13.67%	3.84%	1.81%
	0.25	337	8.55%	2.05%	0.89%
	0.3	234	5.02%	1.02%	0.41%
	0.1	2102	25.12%	8.93%	4.75%
	0.15	934	15.72%	4.64%	2.25%
90	0.2	526	8.99%	2.19%	0.96%
	0.25	337	4.68%	0.93%	0.37%
	0.3	234	2.21%	0.36%	0.13%

Remark 3.1. *When a sample size estimator is matched with a launching rule, a strategy for sample size estimation is defined. In other words, an SSE strategy is based on both a sample size estimator and a launching rule.*

Pointwise sample size estimation strategy. If the launching rule for phase III is $d_n > \delta_{0L}$ and the sample size estimator M_n in (3.5) is applied to estimate M_I, the *Pointwise Strategy* (PWS) is applied.

■ **EXAMPLE 3.3**

Consider, as usual, $\alpha = 2.5\%$ and $1 - \beta = 90\%$. Moreover, let's adopt the simple PWS, whose effect size estimator d_n is obtained when h is the identity function $(h(x) = x)$. With $n = 59$ data per group in phase II (according to Example 3.2) and with $\alpha_{II} = 20\%$, from (3.6) the launch threshold is $\delta_{0L} = z_{80\%}\sqrt{2/59} = 0.155$. When the latter effect size is set as a launch threshold, from (3.7) the maximum sample size is $M_{max} = 875$. More practically, when δ_{0L} is set at 0.15 (as in Situation II of Section I.4.2), then $M_{max} = 934$ (see also Table 3.1).

3.4   Practical aspects of SSE

Different SSE strategies can be adopted, besides the pointwise one. For example, a conservative approach to SSE can be put into practice by plugging into the sample size formula a conservative estimate of δ_t, given by subtracting a certain quantity from the pointwise estimate d_n. Different SSE strategies can present different probabilities of launching phase III and, of course, different sample size estimates.

Before comparing strategies, some important tools for evaluating their performance should be introduced. First, note that the phase III sample size determined on the basis of phase II data (i.e. $M_n^{\bullet}$) can vary, because phase II data vary. Moreover, $M_n^{\bullet}$ contains a certain randomness, since phase II data are random ones: so, it is a random variable. Consequently, the location and the variability parameters (e.g. mean, median, variance, *Mean Square Error* - MSE) of $M_n^{\bullet}$ are of great interest.

Then, note that since phase III is based on the random sample size $M_n^{\bullet}$, its SP becomes a random variable too. The average of this random SP is named *Average Power* (AP) and it is of undoubtable interest.

Consider now that some phase III trials are not launched (due to phase II results), and that not all of those launched resulted significant. Consequently, the overall success probability of the combined phase II *and* phase III trials should be mandatorily taken into account: this is named *Overall Power* (OP). The OP embeds SP of the phase II (i.e. the probability of launching phase III) and the SP of phase III (i.e. the probability of phase III statistical significance).

When the phase III sample size is estimated on the basis of phase II data and when the latter are not included in phase III data to evaluate statistical significance (which is the theoretical framework developed here), the OP is given by the probability to launch multiplied by the AP.

> To conclude, in order to evaluate the performances of SSE strategies, their OPs and MSEs should be considered.

3.4.1   Different SSE strategies

In practical SSE, various strategies, different from the pointwise one (viz. PWS), can be applied. For example, there exists the class of frequentist conservative estimators, and one of its exponents is introduced here.

To motivate the adoption of conservative estimators note first that when d_n falls above δ_t, the pointwise estimator of the sample size results below the ideal M_I, implying that the phase III trial does not achieve the desired SP of $1 - \beta$. In formulas, $d_n > \delta_t$ gives $M_n \leq M_I$. Then, note that, being the distribution of d_n symmetric across δ_t, we have that $P(d_n > \delta_t) = 1/2$ (recall Figure 1.2 in Section 1.1). Consequently, $P(M_n < M_I) = 1/2$. In other words, when the pointwise SSE is applied, phase III trial is underpowered 50% of the time and this rate looks quite high.

Therefore, in order to be conservative, an estimator of δ_t with a lower probability of falling above it can be adopted, and it can be used to compute the sample size as in (3.4). This conservative estimator of the effect size can be obtained by subtracting a certain quantity from d_n.

One standard error conservative SSE strategy. A simple conservative strategy consists in subtracting one standard error of d_n (i.e. $\sigma\sqrt{2/n}$ - see Section 1.2) off the observed value of d_n itself. That is, to consider $d_n^\bullet = d_n - \sigma\sqrt{2/n}$ as an estimator of δ_t (as usual, $\sigma = 1$ is assumed). This estimator can also be viewed as the lower bound of the one-sided confidence interval for δ_t, with $z_\gamma = 1$ (see Section 1.2). This value of z_γ corresponds to the adoption of $\gamma = 84.1\%$. So, let's denote $d_n - \sqrt{2/n}$ with $d_n^{.841}$ and let's call the related sample size estimator $M_n^{.841}$, obtained in accordance with (3.4), the *one standard error conservative sample size estimator*. The SSE strategy which launches phase III when $d_n^{.841} > \delta_{0L}$ and applies $M_n^{.841}$ is called 1SES (i.e. *1 Standard Error Strategy*).

▣   EXAMPLE 3.4

Continuing Example 3.2. The 84.1% conservative estimate of δ_t is $0.48 - \sqrt{2/59} = 0.296$. When $\delta_{0L} = 0.15$ (as in Section 1.4.2) phase III is launched. The sample size estimated by 1SES is, therefore, 240 units per group (i.e. $M_{59}^{.841} = \lfloor 2((1.96 + 1.28)/0.296)^2 \rfloor + 1 = 240$).

Of course, different SSE strategies provide different estimates of sample size. Moreover, given the launch threshold δ_{0L}, different strategies can offer different probabilities to launch phase III; in other words, $P(d_n^\bullet > \delta_{0L})$ depends on the strategy adopted, as described in Wang et al. (2006).

■ **EXAMPLE 3.5**

With $\alpha = 2.5\%$, $1 - \beta = 90\%$ and $\delta_t = 0.5$ the ideal sample size for phase III is $M_I = 85$. Assume that phase III is launched if the effect size estimate overcomes the threshold $\delta_{0L} = 0.145$. In this case the maximum sample size is $M_{\max} = 1000$. Also, consider phase II samples of size $n = 60$. Hence, the probabilities to launch phase III for PWS and 1SES are different, resulting $P(d_{60} > 0.145) = 97.4\%$ and $P(d_{60}^{.841} > 0.145) = 82.8\%$, respectively. It is worth noting that the 1SES strategy, which is built to make the probability of an underpowered trial lower than 50%, on one hand offers an actual underpowering probability of 15.9% (i.e. $1 - 0.841$), but on the other hand it nevertheless presents a probability to launch lower than that of PWS.

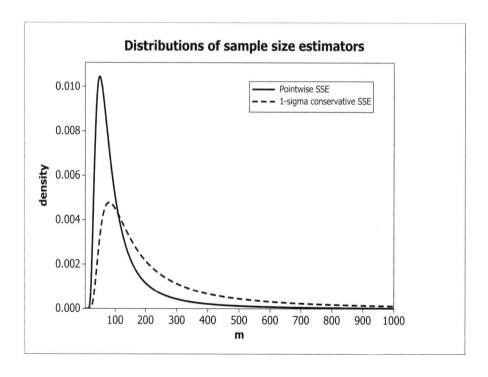

Figure 3.2   *Distributions of the sample size estimators provided by PWS and 1SES with a phase II sample size $n = 60$ (i.e. M_{60} and $M_{60}^{.841}$), obtained with $\alpha = 2.5\%$, $1 - \beta = 90\%$, $\delta_t = 0.5$, and with $\delta_{0L} = 0.145$, giving $M_I = 85$ and $M_{\max} = 1000$.*

3.4.2 The variability in SSE

Focusing on equation (3.2), where the sample size formula $M_n^\bullet$ is based on the random variable $\hat{SP}_n^\bullet(m)$, the latter is the phase III SP with m data estimated with phase II samples of size n. Consequently, $M_n^\bullet$ is a random variable too. Then, $M_n^\bullet$ has a distribution, conditioned by the launching of phase III. Its mean, together with its median and several other indexes regarding its variability, are of interest and can, therefore, be computed. In particular, the mean of sample size estimators is:

$$E[M_n^\bullet | \mathcal{L}] = \sum_m m \, P_{\delta_t}(M_n^\bullet = m \mid \mathcal{L}) \tag{3.8}$$

■ EXAMPLE 3.6

Continuing Example 3.5. In Figure 3.2 the distributions of the sample size estimators PWS and 1SES with $n = 60$ (i.e. M_{60} and $M_{60}^{.841}$) are shown. Note that, although the support of the distribution of $M_n^\bullet$ is discrete, i.e. $\{2, \ldots, 1000\}$, continuous density curves have been drawn because the points of the support are equally spaced. The average of M_{60} is 126, and that of $M_{60}^{.841}$ is 239. Moreover, their medians are 83 and 165, respectively. It can, therefore, be noted that although the pointwise estimator of the effect size d_n is symmetrically distributed around δ_t (and so its median is δ_t), the truncation due to the launch threshold implies that the PWS sample size estimator M_n does not have a median equal to $M_I = 85$.

Thus, the sample size estimators are biased, meaning that their average is not equal to M_I, i.e. the parameter to be estimated. Therefore, in order to evaluate the variability of sample size estimators, the differences of $M_n^\bullet$ from M_I, not from $E[M_n^\bullet | \mathcal{L}]$, should be taken into account. That is, their mean square error (MSE), not their variance, should be computed:

$$MSE[M_n^\bullet | \mathcal{L}] = \sum_m (m - M_I)^2 \, P_{\delta_t}(M_n^\bullet = m \mid \mathcal{L}) \tag{3.9}$$

■ EXAMPLE 3.7

Continuing Example 3.6. The MSEs given by PWS and 1SES in this scenario are 16473 and 41145, respectively, and their square roots resulted 128 and 203. The square root of the MSE represents the mean error of sample size estimators, and it can be compared with sample size estimates. Note that the magnitude of the mean errors is close to that of the sample size to be estimated. This means that the errors are, on average, quite large in this scenario. This fact is quite frequent in SSE. One possibility to reduce the errors of sample size estimators is by increasing the size n of phase II samples.

The actual SP of phase III depends on the random sample size $M_n^\bullet$, so it is a random variable too, which is of undoubtable interest. Formally:

$$SP(M_n^\bullet) = \pi(\alpha, M_n^\bullet, \delta_t)$$

Since $M_n^\bullet$ was based on the estimator of SP (see (3.4)), it results that:

$$SP(M_n^\bullet) = \pi(\alpha, \min\{m \quad \text{such that} \quad \hat{SP}_n^\bullet(m) > 1 - \beta\}, \delta_t)$$

By exploiting the distribution of $M_n^\bullet$, the average of this random SP can be computed, which is named the *Average Power of phase III* (AP) (Wang et al., 2006). In other words, the AP is the mean of the actual SP conditioned on the launching of phase III:

$$AP_n^\bullet = E[SP(M_n^\bullet) \mid \mathcal{L}] = \sum_m SP(m) P_{\delta_t}(M_n^\bullet = m \mid \mathcal{L}) \qquad (3.10)$$

Clearly, the AP depends on the SSE strategy that one adopts and on the size n of phase II samples.

🖥 **EXAMPLE 3.8**

Continuing Examples 3.5 and 3.6. In Figure 3.3 the distributions of $SP(M_{60}^\bullet)$ for PWS and 1SES are shown. Although it might seem that the areas under the curve are not equal (and so at least one of them is not 1), the total probability actually is 1 in both cases. Indeed, the support of $SP(M_n^\bullet)$, beside being discrete, is not uniformly distributed on $(0, 1)$, it is more dense around 90%. Nevertheless, the sum of all single 999 probabilities (i.e. from $SP(2)$ to $SP(1000)$) results 1. The average of $SP(M_{60})$ (i.e. AP_{60}) is 84.4%, and that of $SP(M_{60}^{.841})$ is $AP_{60}^{.841} = 94.7\%$. It can be noted that, since the 1SES tends to provide sample size estimates higher than M_I, the AP of 1SES is higher than $1 - \beta = 90\%$, and also higher than that of PWS. Nevertheless, remember that the probability of the launching of 1SES was somewhat lower than that of PWS.

3.4.3   Overall power and overall type I error

The success probability of the jointed phase II *and* phase III is named Overall Power (OP). This is, in practice, the probability of: succeeding in phase II (i.e. launching phase III) *and* finding statistical significance in phase III.

The theoretical framework where phase II data are not included in phase III ones for testing statistical hypotheses is considered here. In other words, the data of the two phases are not combined. Then, although the launching of phase III, and, eventually,

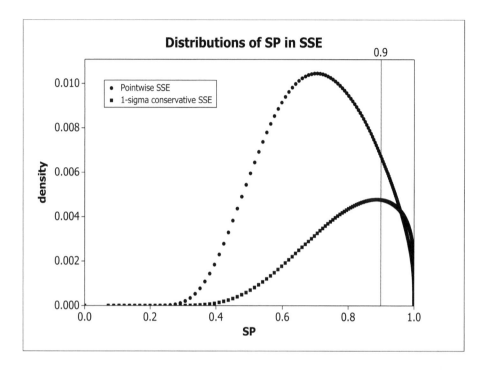

Figure 3.3 *Distributions of the SP provided by PWS and 1SES with $n = 60$, i.e. $SP(M_{60}^{.841})$ and $SP(M_{60})$, with $\alpha = 2.5\%$, $1 - \beta = 90\%$, $\delta_t = 0.5$, and with $\delta_{0L} = 0.145$.*

the estimated sample size of phase III, depends on phase II data, the outcome of phase III does not depend on them (i.e., phase III outcome and phase II data are independent).

Consequently, the OP results from the probability of launching phase III multiplied by the probability of finding statistical significance in phase III, once it has been launched - the multiplication is allowed by the latter independence. The OP is, hence (De Martini, 2011b):

$$OP_n^\bullet = SP_{II} \times AP_n^\bullet = P_{\delta_t}(\mathcal{L}) \times AP_n^\bullet \qquad (3.11)$$

which, thanks to (3.10), becomes:

$$OP_n^\bullet = \sum_m P_{\delta_t}(M_n^\bullet = m)SP(m) \qquad (3.12)$$

Therefore, the OP is always lower than the AP - it is just a bit lower when the launch probability is high.

■ **EXAMPLE 3.9**

> *Continuing Example 3.8. According to (3.11), the OP of the PWS is $97.4\% \times 84.4\% = 82.2\%$, where that of the 1SES is $82.8\% \times 94.7\% = 78.4\%$. Although the OPs are lower than the desired power of 90%, it seems better to adopt the simple PWS, in this specific scenario. On the contrary, if the phase II sample size is increased to $n = 90$, then the analogous probabilities given by (3.11) are: $99.1\% \times 86.0\% = 85.2\%$, and $91.7\% \times 95.3\% = 87.4\%$, for the PWS and 1SES, respectively. That is, the OPs grow and the 1SES seems, in this specific scenario, better than the PWS. It is nevertheless worth noting that the behavior of the sample size estimator should also be evaluated, in particular in terms of mean and MSE.*

When the null hypothesis is true, there is still a probability (higher than zero) of launching phase III and then finding a statistical significance: this is the overall type I error. The latter quantity is given by the product of the levels of the tests of phases II and III, that is: $\alpha_{II} \times \alpha$. In other words, the overall type I error is the OP under the null. When the launching rule is $\mathcal{L}$ iff $d_n^\bullet = h(d_n) > \delta_{0L}$, the phase II type I error results $\alpha_{II} = 1 - \Phi(\sqrt{n/2}\,h^{-1}(\delta_{0L}))$, so that the overall type I error under the null is:

$$OP_{n;0}^\bullet = (1 - \Phi(\sqrt{n/2}\,h^{-1}(\delta_{0L}))) \times \alpha$$

■ **EXAMPLE 3.10**

> *With the same settings of Example 3.5 and $\delta_t = 0$ (i.e. under the null), the probabilities of launching phase III for PWS and 1SES are 21.4% and 3.6%, that correspond to the respective values of $1 - \Phi(\sqrt{n/2}h^{-1}(\delta_{0L}))$ - the function h changes for different effect size estimators. When the level of the phase III test is $\alpha = 2.5\%$, the overall type I errors are 0.5% and 0.1%, for PWS and 1SES.*

3.4.4 Evaluating SSE strategies

For practical purposes, an SSE strategy that has a high launch probability (as close as possible to 1), an AP close to the power $(1 - \beta)$ and a sample size estimator $M_n^\bullet$

close to M_I (that is not just with mean close to M_I, but also with small MSE) would be highly appreciated.

These three features are usually fulfilled by SSE strategies when the information is complete, that is when phase II sample size n tends towards ∞, provided that the launching rule is theoretically satisfied (e.g. the actual effect size δ_t is higher than the launch threshold of clinical relevance δ_{0L}). Moreover, under these conditions the OP tends to $1 - \beta$ when n increases. However, in practice n does not tend to ∞, and it is often lower than the ideal phase III sample M_I. Consequently, the above features cannot be achieved.

Now, note that some of the features are conditional quantities (i.e. AP, mean and MSE of $M_n^\bullet$), whereas some others are not (OP, launch probability). Moreover, some of them regard probabilities, whereas some others concern the behavior of sample size estimators. Many aspects of the sample size estimation strategy should, therefore, be considered. Nevertheless, it would be quite complicated to take all of them into account.

To evaluate the behavior of SSE strategies focus might be placed only on OP and MSE. The former, indeed, embeds launch probability and AP, whereas the latter resumes SSE performances. In practice, an SSE strategy providing a small MSE and an OP close to $1 - \beta$ might be considered a good one, for a reasonable "not too high" phase II sample size. This is also motivated by the fact that an OP close to $1 - \beta$ implies that the AP would be "approximately higher than" $1 - \beta$, which is a good feature from both a conservative statistical perspective and an industrial one.

3.5 Frequentist conservative SSE

> The simple pointwise estimation strategy does not consider the variability implicit in the effect size estimate adopted to determine the sample size. To account for the variability of pilot data (e.g. phase II data) means to be conservative in estimating the sample size. Therefore, this variability should be considered in conservative sample size computation.
>
> An intuitive frequentist technique to be conservative consists in adopting the lower bound of the effect size (computed on the basis of phase II data) to determine the phase III sample size: this is the frequentist approach to conservative SSE (viz. CSSE).
>
> Exact formulas for computing the quantities of interest (e.g. OP, MSE) can be derived by exploiting the distribution of the effect size estimates.

The frequentist technique for CSSE adopts the conservative version of d_n for determining the phase III sample size. This conservative estimator of the effect size consists in the lower bound for δ_t given by the one-sided confidence interval, i.e. $d_n^\gamma = d_n - z_\gamma \sqrt{2/n}$ as in (1.4). The level $\gamma \in (0, 1)$ can be viewed as the *amount of conservativeness*. Thus, from (3.3) and (1.7), the conservative estimator of $SP(m)$ is:

$$\hat{SP}_n^\gamma(m) = \pi(\alpha, m, d_n^\gamma) = \Phi(d_n^\gamma \sqrt{m/2} - z_{1-\alpha})$$

and the consequent γ-*conservative sample size estimator* is:

$$M_n^\gamma = \lfloor 2(z_{1-\alpha} + z_{1-\beta})^2/(d_n^\gamma)^2 \rfloor + 1 \tag{3.13}$$

Frequentist CSSE is based on an effect size estimator which is an increasing function of d_n (i.e. $d_n^\gamma = d_n - z_\gamma \sqrt{2/n} = h(d_n)$, where $h()$ is increasing). Consequently, as shown in Section 3.3, the three launch criteria are equivalent. In order to make the exposition easier, the criterion based on clinical relevance is adopted here: phase III is launched if and only if $d_n^\bullet > \delta_{0L}$ (i.e. $d_n^\gamma > \delta_{0L}$). Consequently, the phase III sample size is allowed to reach, at maximum, $M_{\max}$.

According to (3.8), the mean of the sample size estimator M_n^γ is:

$$E[M_n^\gamma | d_n^\gamma > \delta_{0L}] = \sum_{m=2}^{M_{\max}} m \, P_{\delta_t}(M_n^\gamma = m | d_n^\gamma > \delta_{0L})$$

and, analogously, the MSE in (3.9) becomes:

$$MSE[M_n^\gamma | d_n^\gamma > \delta_{0L}] = \sum_{m=2}^{M_{\max}} (m - M_I)^2 \, P_{\delta_t}(M_n^\gamma = m | d_n^\gamma > \delta_{0L})$$

Now, note that the distribution of M_n^γ can be rebuilt, since:

$$M_n^\gamma = m \quad \text{iff} \quad \lfloor 2(z_{1-\alpha} + z_{1-\beta})^2/(d_n^\gamma)^2 \rfloor = m - 1$$

$$\text{iff} \quad m - 1 \le 2(z_{1-\alpha} + z_{1-\beta})^2/(d_n^\gamma)^2 < m$$

$$\text{iff} \quad \frac{(z_{1-\alpha} + z_{1-\beta})}{\sqrt{m/2}} \le d_n^\gamma < \frac{(z_{1-\alpha} + z_{1-\beta})}{\sqrt{(m-1)/2}}$$

$$\text{iff} \quad \frac{(z_{1-\alpha} + z_{1-\beta})}{\sqrt{m/2}} + z_\gamma \sqrt{2/n} \le d_n < \frac{(z_{1-\alpha} + z_{1-\beta})}{\sqrt{(m-1)/2}} + z_\gamma \sqrt{2/n}$$

Now, on the basis of the distribution of d_n, which is $N(\delta_t, 2/n)$:

$$P_{\delta_t}(M_n^\gamma = m) =$$

$$\Phi\left(\sqrt{\frac{n}{2}}\left(\frac{z_{1-\alpha} + z_{1-\beta}}{\sqrt{(m-1)/2}} - \delta_t\right) + z_\gamma\right) - \Phi\left(\sqrt{\frac{n}{2}}\left(\frac{z_{1-\alpha} + z_{1-\beta}}{\sqrt{m/2}} - \delta_t\right) + z_\gamma\right)$$

$$\tag{3.14}$$

The conditional distribution of M_n^γ can be rewritten in light of the above formula and on the probability of launching, that is $P(d_n^\gamma > \delta_{0L}) = \Phi(\sqrt{\frac{n}{2}}(\delta_t - \delta_{0L}) - z_\gamma)$. So:

$$P_{\delta_t}(M_n^\gamma = m | d_n^\gamma > \delta_{0L}) = \left[\Phi\left(\sqrt{\frac{n}{2}}\left(\frac{z_{1-\alpha} + z_{1-\beta}}{\sqrt{(m-1)/2}} - \delta_t \right) + z_\gamma \right) \right.$$

$$\left. - \Phi\left(\sqrt{\frac{n}{2}}\left(\frac{z_{1-\alpha} + z_{1-\beta}}{\sqrt{m/2}} - \delta_t \right) + z_\gamma \right) \right] \Big/ \Phi\left(\sqrt{\frac{n}{2}}(\delta_t - \delta_{0L}) - z_\gamma \right) \quad (3.15)$$

that can be used to rewrite the conditional mean and MSE above, and also the AP and the OP. To focus on AP and OP, recall that $SP(m) = \Phi(\delta_t\sqrt{m/2} - z_{1-\alpha})$. Then, the AP in (3.10) assumes, for frequentist CSSE and thanks to (3.15), the following formulation:

$$AP_n^\gamma = \sum_{m=2}^{M_{\max}} \left[\Phi\left(\sqrt{\frac{n}{2}}\left(\frac{z_{1-\alpha} + z_{1-\beta}}{\sqrt{(m-1)/2}} - \delta_t \right) + z_\gamma \right) \right.$$

$$\left. - \Phi\left(\sqrt{\frac{n}{2}}\left(\frac{z_{1-\alpha} + z_{1-\beta}}{\sqrt{m/2}} - \delta_t \right) + z_\gamma \right) \right] \times \frac{\Phi(\delta_t\sqrt{m/2} - z_{1-\alpha})}{\Phi(\sqrt{\frac{n}{2}}(\delta_t - \delta_{0L}) - z_\gamma)} \quad (3.16)$$

The OP, according to (3.12), is simplified in the following:

$$OP_n(\gamma) = \sum_{m=2}^{M_{\max}} \left[\Phi\left(\sqrt{\frac{n}{2}}\left(\frac{z_{1-\alpha} + z_{1-\beta}}{\sqrt{(m-1)/2}} - \delta_t \right) + z_\gamma \right) \right.$$

$$\left. - \Phi\left(\sqrt{\frac{n}{2}}\left(\frac{z_{1-\alpha} + z_{1-\beta}}{\sqrt{m/2}} - \delta_t \right) + z_\gamma \right) \right] \times \Phi(\delta_t\sqrt{m/2} - z_{1-\alpha}) \quad (3.17)$$

These formulas have been used to compute Examples 3.6-9. The notation $OP_n(\gamma)$ is used, instead of OP_n^γ, to emphasize that the OP under the γ-conservative approach is a function of γ. For γ values defining specific strategies, $OP_n^\bullet$ can also be used (e.g. OP_n^{1SES} with $\gamma = 84.1\%$).

For completeness, the conditional mean and MSE of the sample size are:

$$E[M_n^\gamma | d_n^\gamma > \delta_{0L}] = \sum_{m=2}^{M_{\max}} m \left[\Phi\left(\sqrt{\frac{n}{2}}\left(\frac{z_{1-\alpha} + z_{1-\beta}}{\sqrt{(m-1)/2}} - \delta_t \right) + z_\gamma \right) \right.$$

$$\left. - \Phi\left(\sqrt{\frac{n}{2}}\left(\frac{z_{1-\alpha} + z_{1-\beta}}{\sqrt{m/2}} - \delta_t \right) + z_\gamma \right) \right] \Big/ \Phi\left(\sqrt{\frac{n}{2}}(\delta_t - \delta_{0L}) - z_\gamma \right) \quad (3.18)$$

and

$$MSE[M_n^\gamma | d_n^\gamma > \delta_{0L}] = \sum_{m=2}^{M_{\max}} (m - M_I)^2 \left[\Phi \left(\sqrt{\frac{n}{2}} \left(\frac{z_{1-\alpha} + z_{1-\beta}}{\sqrt{(m-1)/2}} - \delta_t \right) + z_\gamma \right) \right.$$

$$\left. - \Phi \left(\sqrt{\frac{n}{2}} \left(\frac{z_{1-\alpha} + z_{1-\beta}}{\sqrt{m/2}} - \delta_t \right) + z_\gamma \right) \right] \bigg/ \Phi \left(\sqrt{\frac{n}{2}} (\delta_t - \delta_{0L}) - z_\gamma \right) \quad (3.19)$$

The generic γ-conservative SSE strategy adopts M_n^γ and launches phase III only when $d_n^\gamma > \delta_{0L}$. When $\gamma = 84.1\%$ is adopted, the 1SES conservative strategy arises (see Section 3.4.1). With $\gamma = 50\%$ the simple PWS strategy is put into practice (Section 3.3.1).

Remember that with PWS the probability that the phase III trial is underpowered (i.e. that $M_n \leq M_I$, unconditionally on the launch) is $1/2$, which looks quite high. If, in order to be conservative, one wants to reduce the latter probability to $1/k$ (with $k > 2$), it is sufficient to adopt $\gamma = 1 - 1/k$.

Third quartile CSSE strategy. Setting $k = 4$, $M_n^{.75}$ is applied to estimate the sample size: this is the so-called *third quartile conservative strategy* (3QS), which launches phase III only when $d_n^{.75} > \delta_{0L}$. Note that in this case there is actually a 25% probability to be underpowered in phase III, i.e. $P(M_n^{.75} \leq M_I) = 0.25$.

3.6 Optimal frequentist CSSE

It is intuitive that the more conservative a frequentist CSSE approach is (i.e. the higher the amount of conservative γ is set) the lower the probability to launch and the higher the Average Power of phase III are. On the contrary, the less conservative it is (i.e. the lower γ is) the higher the probability to launch and the lower the Average Power of phase III.

Since the Overall Power is the product of the two quantities above (i.e. the probability to launch and the Average Power), to evaluate it as a function of γ is a direct consequence. This is mainly in order to find convenient values of γ, which are those providing high values of the OP.

It should, at first, be remarked that extreme γ values (i.e. close to 0 or 1) give very small OP values, actually close to zero. Then, this implies that there exists an intermediate amount of conservativeness, say γ^O, that gives an OP maximum: let's call this γ^O the *Optimal* γ.

If γ^O is known, it would be certainly adopted, but in practice it is unknown since it depends on the unknown effect size δ_t. Nevertheless, pilot data can be used to estimate this optimal γ, and the related conservative sample size can then be computed on the basis of the estimated optimal amount of conservativeness: this strategy for CSSE is the *Calibrated Optimal Strategy* (COS).

3.6.1 Optimal conservativeness

First, the $OP_n(\gamma)$ in (3.17) is a continuous positive function of γ. From (3.17) it is easy to obtain that the limits of the OP for the extreme values of γ are 0:

$$\lim_{\gamma \to 0^+} OP_n(\gamma) = \lim_{\gamma \to 1^-} OP_n(\gamma) = 0$$

Consequently, $OP_n(\gamma)$ has a maximum in $(0, 1)$, and it is called γ'_n. Formally, the argmax of $OP_n(\gamma)$ is γ'_n. To compute the maximum analytically presents some technical difficulties, especially in deriving a composite function of the standard normal distribution. Then, the problem is approached numerically.

■ **EXAMPLE 3.11**

Like in Example 3.5, $\alpha = 2.5\%$, $1 - \beta = 90\%$ and $\delta_t = 0.5$ were set, so that $M_I = 85$. The launching rule is $d_n^\gamma > \delta_{0L} = 0.145$, implying $M_{\max} = 1000$. In order to consider a size of the phase II sample around M_I (in particular from $M_I/3$ to $4M_I/3$, approximately) $n = 30, 60, 90$ and 120 is set. The OP is computed and reported in Figure 3.4. First, it is easy to see that the OP function is a concave one. When $n = 60$, then $argmax\,OP_{60}(\gamma) = \gamma'_{60} = 0.649$, and the maximum OP is $OP_{60}(0.649) = 0.840$. If, in this case, the 1SES were to be adopted, then the OP would be lower: $OP_{60}(0.841) = OP_{60}^{1SES} = 0.783$. Note that the optimal γ'_n depends on n, and that γ'_n increases as n grows. Indeed, $argmax\,OP_{120}(\gamma) = \gamma'_{120} = 0.805$. Note also that the maximum OP can be even higher than 90%: $OP_{120}(0.805) = 0.919$. Moreover, γ'_n depends on δ_t, α and β. For example, when $\delta_t = 0.4$ and with the same type I error and power, then $\gamma'_{60} = 0.527$, and $OP_{60}(0.527) = 0.750$.

From Figure 3.4 it can be noted that γ'_n seems to tend to 1 as n tends to ∞, but this behavior of $OP_n(\gamma)$ will not be studied here because it is not of main interest in this practical context. Indeed, it is better to focus on the fact that $OP_n(\gamma'_n)$ can be higher than $1 - \beta$. In this case, when γ'_n is assumed as the conservative amount to be applied (i.e. M_I is estimated through $M_n^{\gamma'_n}$) the CSSE strategy is more powerful than requested (in accordance with the discussion on SSE features of Section 3.4.4) and the MSE turns out to be unnecessarily large.

Consequently, let us consider a good CSSE strategy (i.e. a good amount of conservativeness γ) the one providing the maximum possible OP when this maximum is lower than, or equal to, the prefixed power (i.e. when $OP_n(\gamma'_n) \leq 1 - \beta$), and an OP equal to the power $1 - \beta$ when the maximum OP exceeds the latter threshold. In

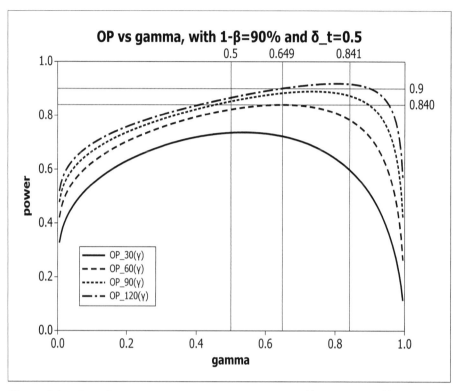

Figure 3.4   *Overall Power as a function of γ, with $\alpha = 2.5\%$, $1 - \beta = 90\%$, $\delta_t = 0.5$, $\delta_{0L} = 0.145$ and with phase II sample size $n = 30, 60, 90$ and 120.*

the latter circumstance, being $OP_n(\gamma)$ a concave function of γ, there are two roots of the equation $OP_n(\gamma) = 1 - \beta$. In other words, if the roots are defined as $\gamma_{n,1}$ and $\gamma_{n,2}$, with $\gamma_{n,1} < \gamma_{n,2}$:

$$OP_n(\gamma_{n,1}) = OP_n(\gamma_{n,2}) = 1 - \beta < OP_n(\gamma'_n)$$

Now, note that the less conservative solution (i.e. $\gamma_{n,1}$) provides a lower sample size with respect to $\gamma_{n,2}$, and it is, therefore, preferable. Then, the best choice for γ is $\gamma_{n,1}$ since this provides both the desired OP and the lowest sample size. The optimal amount of conservativeness, γ_n^O, is therefore defined:

$$\gamma_n^O = \begin{cases} \gamma'_n & \text{if} \quad OP_n(\gamma'_n) \leq 1 - \beta \\ \gamma_{n,1} & \text{if} \quad OP_n(\gamma'_n) > 1 - \beta \end{cases} \tag{3.20}$$

■ **EXAMPLE 3.12**

Continuing Example 3.11. With $n = 120$, $\gamma'_{120} = 0.805$ and $OP_{120}(0.805) = 0.919$ were obtained. In this scenario, the first root of the equation $OP_{120}(\gamma) = 0.9$ is $\gamma_{120,1} = 0.645$. So, the definition (3.20) gives $\gamma^O_{120} = 0.645$. The average sample size and the MSE given by the optimal choice of conservativeness γ^O_{120} (i.e. those provided by $M^{0.645}_{120}$) are 136 and 14674 (the mean error, i.e. the square root of MSE, is 121). These results are better than those provided by adopting $\gamma'_{120} = 0.805$, that are 185 and 31932 (179).

From Figure 3.4 it can be noted that the OP increases as n grows (i.e. $OP_n(\gamma) < OP_{n'}(\gamma)$ if $n < n'$). This implies that the maximum of the OP also increases and, more importantly, that the intersection of $OP_n(\gamma)$ with $1 - \beta$ (i.e. the optimal amount of conservativeness $\gamma_{n,1}$) decreases, becoming closer to 50%. Consequently, also the constrained optimum γ, i.e. γ^O_n, tends to 50%. This will not be proved analytically, so the behavior of γ^O_n is just shown in Figure 3.5. It is worth noting that the limit of γ^O_n towards 50% means that the asymptotically optimal conservative strategy is that with $\gamma = 50\%$, i.e. the PWS. This result is also intuitive: as the information increases there is less need to be conservative.

3.6.2 The Calibrated Optimal Strategy (COS)

The size n of the experimental pilot samples is, of course, finite, and in clinical trials the size of the phase II sample is often not greater than the optimal phase III sample size M_I. Consequently, the optimal amount of conservativeness γ^O_n is often different from 50%; it is also unknown, since it depends on δ_t. Phase II data can, therefore, be used not only to estimate M_I but, in advance, to estimate γ^O_n. The latter parameter can be estimated by, say, g^O_n and then $M^{g^O_n}_n$ can be adopted for estimating M_I (De Martini, 2011b). This is an application of the well known technique of *Calibration*, which was introduced by Hall and Martin (1988); see also Efron and Tibshirani (2003).

Let us now define this calibrated CSSE strategy. First, it is launched if $d_n > \delta_{0L}$, as the PWS is. Here, $OP_n(\gamma)$ is estimated by plugging d_n in place of δ_t into equation (3.17), obtaining $\hat{OP}_n(\gamma)$. The argmax of $\hat{OP}_n(\gamma)$ is g'_n, in analogy with γ'_n. Then, the estimated constrained optimal γ (namely g^O_n) is derived from $\hat{OP}_n(\gamma)$ in analogy with (3.20), and so it is:

$$g^O_n = \begin{cases} g'_n & \text{if} \quad \hat{OP}_n(g'_n) \leq 1 - \beta \\ g_{n,1} & \text{if} \quad \hat{OP}_n(g'_n) > 1 - \beta \end{cases} \tag{3.21}$$

where $g_{n,1}$ is defined, in analogy with $\gamma_{n,1}$, just if $\hat{OP}_n(g'_n) > 1 - \beta$.

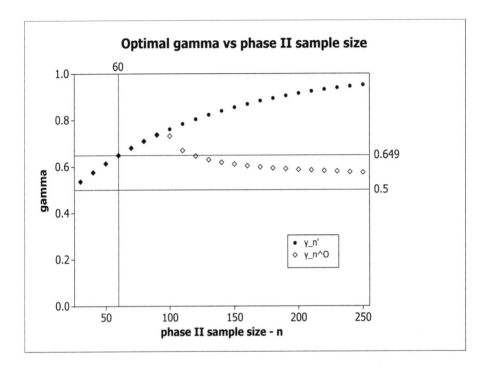

Figure 3.5   *Optimal and constrained optimal γ (i.e. γ'_n and γ^O_n), with $\alpha = 2.5\%$, $1 - \beta =$ 90%, $\delta_t = 0.5$, $\delta_{0L} = 0.145$ and with $n = 30, \ldots, 250$. It is remarked that $\gamma'_{60} = 0.649$, in accordance with Figure 3.4.*

So, the calibrated optimal effect size estimator is $d_n^{g_n^O}$, which provides its related g_n^O-conservative sample size estimator $M_n^{g_n^O}$: this is the *Calibrated Optimal CSSE Strategy*, namely COS.

■ **EXAMPLE 3.13**

> *In the same scenario of Example 3.5, that is $\alpha = 2.5\%$, $1 - \beta = 90\%$, $\delta_t = 0.5$ and $\delta_{0L} = 0.145$, so that $M_I = 85$ and $M_{\max} = 1000$, the COS provides an AP of 89.7%, an OP of 87.4%, an average sample size of 115 and a MSE of 3657 (mean error 61). This performance is evidently better than those provided by PWS and 1SES. In Table 3.2 the most important features of these CSSE strategies, together with those of 3QS, are reported in order to allow comparison.*

Table 3.2   Average power, launch probability, overall power, mean and MSE of the sample size estimators of four CSSE strategies (viz. PWS, 3QS, 1SES, and COS), with $\alpha = 2.5\%$, $1 - \beta = 90\%$, $\delta_t = 0.5$, $\delta_{0L} = 0.145$ and $n = 60$.

	γ	$AP_{60}^{\bullet}$	$P(\mathcal{L})$	$OP_{60}^{\bullet}$	$E[M_{60}^{\bullet}|\mathcal{L}]$	$MSE[M_{60}^{\bullet}|\mathcal{L}]$
PWS	50%	84.5%	97.4%	82.4%	126	18443
3QS	75%	92.2%	89.7%	82.7%	198	45325
1SES	84.1%	94.7%	82.8%	78.3%	239	64883
COS	g_{60}^{O}	89.7%	97.4%	87.4%	115	3657

A wide comparison among CSSE strategies in many different scenarios will be shown later, in Section 3.8.

3.6.3   How COS works

In order to explain the better performance of COS the behavior of its components is illustrated in detail. First, let's consider the estimators of the sample size. In Figure 3.6 the sample size estimates M_{60}, $M_{60}^{.841}$ and $M_{60}^{g_n^O}$ as a function of the effect size estimate d_{60} are shown. Note that the estimates provided by COS are much more condensed around $M_I = 85$ than those of PWS and 1SES; moreover, their maximum, given by the minimum acceptable estimate of δ_t (i.e. 0.145), is just 266, not 1000 as PWS and 1SES provide.

The reason for this behavior of COS sample size estimator can be attributed to the relationship between the estimated optimum γ, i.e. g_{60}^{O}, and the observed effect size d_{60}. In Figure 3.7 this relationship is shown (for completeness, also g_{60}' is reported). In detail, for small d_{60}s, that are those usually providing high sample size estimates, the COS provides low γs, even lower than 50% (in particular for $d_{60} < 0.378$), so that $d_{60}^{g_{60}^O} > d_{60}$ and COS sample size estimates are much lower than $M_{\max}$. In practice, the COS indicates that when the probability of launching is low (i.e. d_{60} is close to δ_{0L}) the maximum of the OP is obtained with a low γ. For central and high values of d_{60}, comparable values of the effect size are indicated by COS's $d_{60}^{g_{60}^O}$, since g_{60}^{O} is not far from 50%. Note also that with $d_{60} \geq 0.602$ the estimated OP exceeds the power and consequently $g_{60}^{O} = g_{60,1}$.

3.7   Bayesian CSSE

Another CSSE technique is based on the consideration of the Bayesian posterior distribution of the effect size δ_t instead of an estimate of the latter, as has been adopted until now.

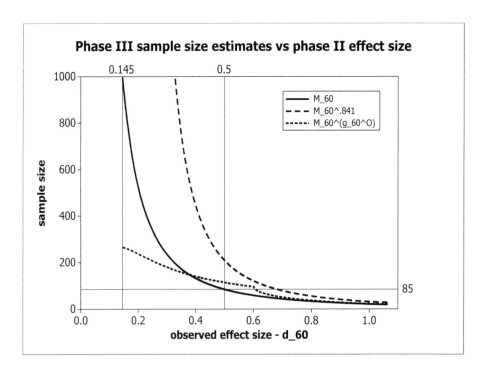

Figure 3.6   *Sample size estimates of PWS, 1SES and COS vs d_n, with $\alpha = 2.5\%$, $1 - \beta = 90\%$, $\delta_t = 0.5$, $\delta_{0L} = 0.145$ and with $n = 60$.*

In other words, a probability mass is put around the observed phase II effect size, and, consequently, the averaged SP is computed at a given sample size, giving the Bayesian estimate of the SP. Then, the minimum sample size whose Bayesian SP exceeds the prefixed power is the Bayesian sample size estimate of M_I.

Since the sample size estimate given by this Bayesian approach can not be limited, and can therefore be higher than $M_{\max}$, a Bayesian truncated strategy whose maximum sample size estimate is $M_{\max}$ is also introduced.

From the Bayesian perspective, the estimation of δ_t is based on its posterior distribution, depending on the observed phase II data and on a certain prior distribution. A simple solution, which is also often adopted, consists in assuming a noninformative

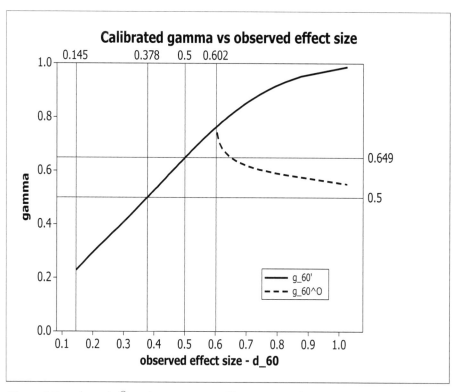

Figure 3.7 g'_{60} and g^O_{60} vs d_n, with $\alpha = 2.5\%$, $1 - \beta = 90\%$, $\delta_t = 0.5$, $\delta_{0L} = 0.145$ and with $n = 60$.

prior which gives:

$$d^\bullet_n = \delta^{post}_t \sim N(d_n, 2/n)$$

Then, the Bayesian posterior SP (i.e. $\pi(\alpha, m, \delta^{post}_t)$) assumes a certain distribution, and its average is considered to be the Bayesian estimator of the SP (see, for example Chuang-Stein, 2006):

$$\hat{SP}^{Bas}_n(m) = \int_{-\infty}^{+\infty} \pi(\alpha, m, z)\, d\Phi_{d_n, 2/n}(z) \tag{3.22}$$

From (3.2) we then have:

$$M^{Bas}_n = \min\{m \quad \text{such that} \quad \hat{SP}^{Bas}_n(m) > 1 - \beta\}$$

Now, note that $\lim_{m \to \infty} \hat{SP}_n^{Bas}(m) = \Phi(d_n \sqrt{n/2})$, so that in some circumstances this limit can be lower than $1 - \beta$, and consequently M_n^{Bas} does not exist. In particular, the probability of this event is $P(\Phi(d_n \sqrt{n/2}) < 1 - \beta)) = \Phi(z_{1-\beta} - \delta_t \sqrt{n/2})$. Moreover, in other circumstances M_n^{Bas} can be simply higher than $M_{\max}$. Consequently, in order to provide a limited version of Bayesian sample size estimation the *Bayesian truncated estimator* is introduced:

$$M_n^{BaT} = \min\{M_n^{Bas}, M_{\max}\}$$

Bayesian and truncated Bayesian CSSE strategies. The strategies applying the sample size estimators M_n^{Bas} and M_n^{BaT} and whose launching rule is based only on the point estimator only and coincides with that of PWS (i.e. $\mathcal{L}$ iff $d_n > \delta_{0L}$), are named *Bayesian Strategy* (BAS) and *Bayesian Truncated strategy* (BAT), respectively.

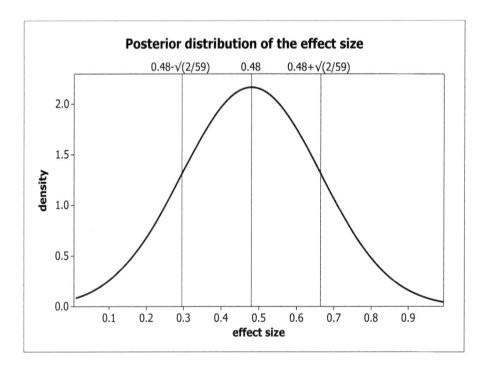

Figure 3.8   *Posterior distribution of δ with $d_{59} = 0.48$, that is $\delta_t^{post} \sim N(0.48, \sqrt{2/59})$.*

■ **EXAMPLE 3.14**

Continuing Examples 3.2 and 3.4. By adopting the Bayesian approach in CSSE, note first that the classical sample size estimate is finite, since $\lim_{m\to\infty} \hat{SP}_n^{Bas}(m)$
$= \Phi(0.48\sqrt{59/2}) = 99.5\% > 90\%$. *Then, the posterior distribution of the effect size should be considered, i.e.* $\delta_t^{post} \sim N(0.48, \sqrt{2/59})$, *and it is reported in Figure 3.8. Now, from (3.22) we have that* $\hat{SP}_{59}^{Bas}(M_{\max}) = \hat{SP}_{59}^{Bas}(934) > 90\%$, *so that not only is the Bayesian estimate finite, but* $M_{59}^{Bas} < 934$ *is also obtained. In particular, once again from (3.22) some SP estimates resulted:* $\hat{SP}_{59}^{Bas}(100) = 80.80\%$, $\hat{SP}_{59}^{Bas}(150) = 87.83\%$. *The Bayesian SP estimates, together with those of PWS and of 1SES of Examples 3.2 and 3.4, are reported in Figure 3.9, where it can be viewed that* $M_{59}^{Bas} = M_{59}^{BaT} = 178$.

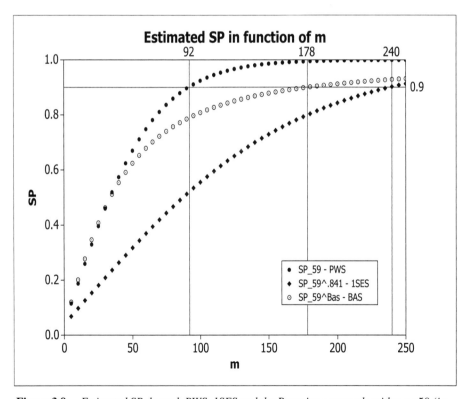

Figure 3.9 *Estimated SP through PWS, 1SES and the Bayesian approach, with* $n = 59$ *(i.e.* $\hat{SP}_{59}(m)$, $\hat{SP}_{59}^{84.1\%}(m)$ *and* $\hat{SP}_{59}^{Bas}(m)$*), vs the phase III sample size m, with* $d_{59} = 0.48$ *and* $\alpha = 2.5\%$.

It is interesting to note that the frequentist and the Bayesian approaches to SP estimation are related. One could, indeed, think about the possibility of averaging the frequentist conservative SP estimators over some different amounts of conservativeness. That is, for example, to estimate $SP(m)$ through $\sum_{i=1}^{9} \hat{SP}_n^{i/10}/9$, i.e. the average over $\gamma = 0.1, 0.2, \ldots, 0.9$. By extending the latter average over the whole set of possible γs, i.e. $\gamma \in (0,1)$, the average becomes an integral which, through a change of variable, coincides with the Bayesian estimator of the SP:

$$\int_0^1 \hat{SP}_n^\gamma(m)d\gamma = \int_{-\infty}^{+\infty} \pi(\alpha, m, z)\, d\Phi_{d_n,2/n}(z) = \hat{SP}_n^{Bas}(m) \qquad (3.23)$$

This equation will be useful for Bayesian CSSE in both a general parametric and a general nonparametric frameworks (see Chapters 5 and 9).

As it concerns the mean and MSE of M_n^{Bas} and M_n^{BaT} and the OP of the respective strategies, formulas (3.8), (3.9) and (3.12) should be applied. The computation can be performed numerically, not analytically as for the γ-conservative strategies of Section 3.5.

3.8   A comparison of CSSE strategies

The CSSE strategies introduced in previous Sections (viz. PWS, 1SES, 3QS, COS, BAS and BAT) are compared here under many different settings. In any of the cases considered, the effect size of phase II is equal to that of phase III (namely Scenario 1). The results are evaluated in terms of overall power (OP) and of sample size estimates behavior.

Although Bayesian techniques provide good OP, they show very high averaged sample size estimates; principally, the variability in estimation is so high that Bayesian sample size estimation cannot be recommended for practical purposes.

The frequentist conservative SSE strategies 1SES and 3QS suffer in terms of OP (due to low launch probabilities) when the phase II sample size n is lower than the ideal M_I of phase III; moreover, they present quite a large variability in sample size estimation.

COS provides the best performances, being its OP close to the prefixed power and being its MSE clearly the lowest. The gain of COS with respect to PWS in terms of OP is about 3%; since it concerns sample size estimates, those provided by PWS are (approximately) 50% more biased than those provided by COS, and with a mean error (approximately) 100% larger. By adopting COS, therefore, the overall success probability increases and costs and experimental times are considerably reduced and standardized.

In general, the phase II sample size should not be chosen to be too small (e.g. $n \approx M_I/3$): a pilot sample size around M_I is strongly recommended (i.e. $2M_I/3 \leq n \leq 4M_I/3$); the launch threshold (δ_{0L}) should be set lower than one half of the true effect size δ_t, better if $\delta_{0L} \approx \delta_t/3$; the OP often results a bit lower than the power, so that $1 - \beta = 90\%$ should be preferred to 80%. These suggestions can be seen as *operating conditions* of CSSE.

3.8.1 Study design and comparison tools

CSSE strategies are evaluated considering that the effect sizes of phases II and III are equal, namely in Scenario 1. In the following Chapter the possibility that they differ is allowed for, and some new Scenarios will be considered.

To study CSSE strategies, the parameters are set as follows: $\alpha = 2.5\%$, $1 - \beta = 80\%, 90\%$, $\delta_t = 0.2, 0.5, 0.8$, $\delta_{0L} = 0.1, 0.25$. Note that ten settings (i.e. 2 power levels times 3 δ_ts with $\delta_{0L} = 0.1$ plus 2 power levels times 2 δ_ts with $\delta_{0L} = 0.25$) have been built, and there exists a different ideal sample size M_I for each setting. Then, the behavior of the six strategies for 12 values of n, from $n = M_I/3$ to $n = 4M_I$ with step $M_I/3$, is evaluated. Small values of n, from $M_I/3$ to $4M_I/3$, are considered important from a practical standpoint, whereas higher ones are useful to study the asymptotic behavior of CSSE strategies.

According to Section 3.4.4, in order to evaluate the global behavior of the strategies, the overall SP of phases II and III (i.e. OP) is considered. Moreover, for evaluating sample size estimator distributions, conditional to launching, the average of the sample size estimators together with their MSE is computed.

3.8.2 Results

As the pilot sample size n increases, the CSSE strategies are consistent: the OP tends to $1 - \beta$ and the sample size estimators here considered tend to M_I (see Figures 3.10, 3.11, 3.12, 3.13, 3.14, 3.15). This fact can also be proved analytically.

In general, with $n = M_I/3$ all methods perform poorly, providing either low OPs or very high averaged sample sizes and MSEs. So, $2M_I/3 \leq n \leq 4M_I/3$ is considered for comparing performances. Moreover, all strategies suffer when the true effect size δ_t is close to the launch threshold (δ_{0L}): it would be better to set $\delta_{0L} \approx \delta_t/3$. Furthermore, the OP often results a bit lower than the power and, consequently, $1 - \beta = 90\%$ is preferred to 80%.

Regarding Bayesian strategies, although their OP is good (being close to the power), they present very high mean and MSE of sample size estimators. Since BAT exploits its upper limit $M_{\max}$, its mean and MSE are lower than those of BAS. Nevertheless, the sample size estimator M_n^{BaT} still presents a very large variability, besides a high mean: on average (over the 30 different performances given by three ns times the ten

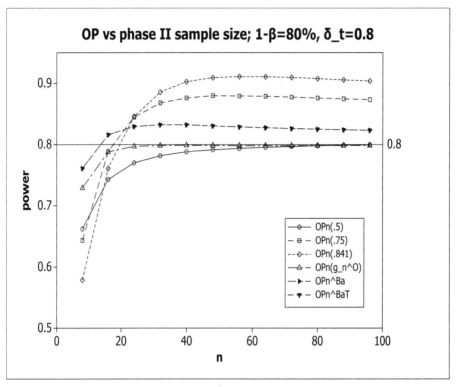

Figure 3.10   *Overall Power of CSSE strategies, with* $\alpha = 2.5\%$ *and* $\delta_{0L} = 0.1$, $1 - \beta = 80\%$, $\delta_t = 0.8$.

settings) its mean error (i.e the square root of MSE) is approximately 6 times higher than that of $M_n^{g_n^O}$; moreover, its mean is more than twice that of COS.

Among the four remaining strategies, COS provides, on average, an OP which is the closest to $1 - \beta$, and also the highest. In particular, the distances of OPs of PWS, 3QS, and 1SES from $1 - \beta$ are higher than those of COS with a factor of 3.5, 3.1 and 4.4, respectively; in particular, the absolute gains in power of COS with respect to PWS, 3QS, and 1SES are 2.9%, 2.1%, and 5.8%, respectively.

COS sample size estimator provides therefore better results than the other three CSSE strategies: it is less biased and shows a lower MSE. In particular, PWS, 3QS, and 1SES increase the bias from M_I (i.e. $|E[M_n^{\bullet}] - M_I|$), with respect to COS, with factors of 1.5, 4.8 and 6.6, respectively (the average of the rates between the bias from M_I has been computed). The factors of the increase of mean error given by PWS, 3QS, and 1SES with respect to COS are 2.1, 3.3 and 4.0, respectively.

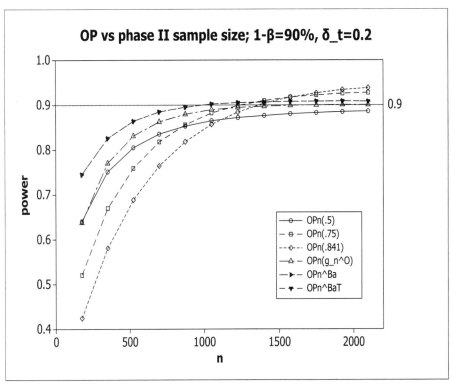

Figure 3.11   *Overall Power of CSSE strategies, with* $\alpha = 2.5\%$ *and* $\delta_{0L} = 0.1$, $1 - \beta = 90\%$, $\delta_t = 0.2$.

To conclude, thanks to the behavior if its sample size estimator, COS reduces costs and times of the experiment and improves the success probability of the two phases jointly (i.e. the OP). Moreover, by adopting COS the variability in SSE is considerably reduced.

3.9   Discussing Situations I and II in Section I.4

Let's start with Situation II in I.4.2. In previous Examples 3.2, 3.4 and 3.14, the sample size estimates given by PWS, 1SES and BAS/BAT were provided, resulting 92, 240 and 178, respectively. As anticipated during the exposition of Situation II, the estimated effect size is $0.3558 = 0.48 - z_{0.75}/\sqrt{59/2}$ with 3QS application, so that $M_{59}^{.75}$, according to (3.13), results 166.

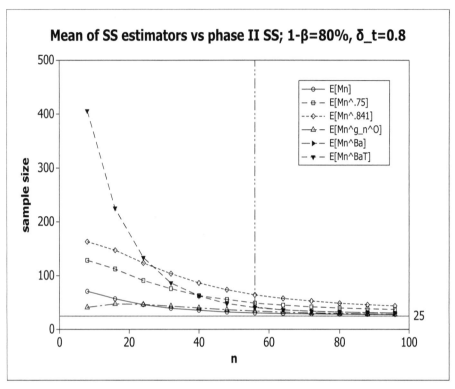

Figure 3.12   *Mean of sample size estimators of the strategies, with $\alpha = 2.5\%$ and $\delta_{0L} = 0.1$, $1 - \beta = 80\%$, $\delta_t = 0.8$.*

In light of the results of the previous Section, the sample size given by COS is the most affordable. Settings $\delta_{0L} = 0.15$ as in Situation II, and given $d_{59} = 0.48$, the estimated overall power $\widehat{OP}_{59}(\gamma)$ is illustrated in Figure 3.16. Then, the estimate of the optimal level of conservativeness results $g_{59}^{O} = 61.3\%$. Consequently, the optimal conservative effect size estimate is $0.48 - z_{0.613}/\sqrt{59/2} = 0.427$. Thus, the COS estimate of the sample size is $M_{59}^{g_{59}^{O}} = 116$, using (3.13).

As far as Situation I in I.4.1 is concerned, it is shown in Section 2.7 and 2.8 that p-values of $1\% - 3\%$ do not provide a reproducibility probability high enough for giving stability, and so omit the second pivotal trial. As a consequence, a new confirmative trial should be run, or should not be stopped if it has already commenced.

Indeed, the two phase III trials are often run parallel in order to speed up the development of clinical research. If this is not so, data from the first phase III can be added to those of phase II for estimating the SP and then for planning the subsequent phase

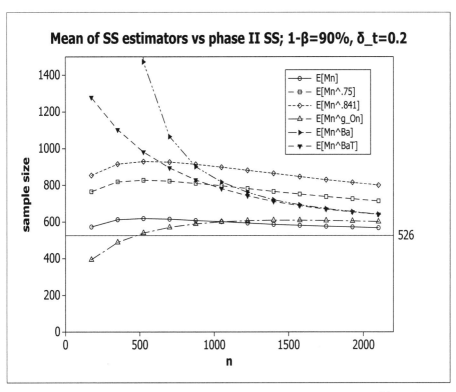

Figure 3.13 *Mean of sample size estimators of the strategies, with* $\alpha = 2.5\%$ *and* $\delta_{0L} = 0.1$, $1 - \beta = 90\%$, $\delta_t = 0.2$.

III. The conservative techniques for SSE presented in this Chapter can therefore be adopted.

3.10 Sample size estimation for the two-tailed setting

In the two-tailed setting, sample size estimation is performed in analogy with the one-tailed test, but the type I error probability α is divided by two. This is due to the definition of the two-tailed SP of Section 1.7.

The ideal sample size is then easily derived, together with the conservative sample size estimates of different strategies. The results of the strategy comparison in Section 3.8 remain valid also for the two-tailed setting.

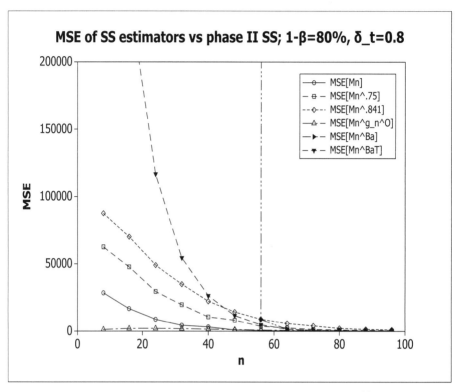

Figure 3.14   *MSE of sample size estimators of the strategies, with $\alpha = 2.5\%$ and $\delta_{0L} = 0.1$, $1 - \beta = 80\%$, $\delta_t = 0.8$.*

Let us first consider the SP of the two-tailed test in (1.15), and denote it by $SP_2(m)$, according to the definition of $SP(m)$ in Section 3.1. Then, the *ideal* sample size, in analogy with (3.1), is:

$$M_{2,I} = \min\{m \quad \text{such that} \quad SP_2(m) > 1-\beta\} = \lfloor 2(z_{1-\alpha/2}+z_{1-\beta})^2/(\delta_t)^2 \rfloor +1 \tag{3.24}$$

Being $\hat{SP}^{\bullet}_{2;n}(m)$ a generic estimator of $SP_2(m)$ based on samples of size n, the generic sample size estimator is obtained:

$$M^{\bullet}_{2,n} = \min\{m \quad \text{such that} \quad \hat{SP}^{\bullet}_{2;n}(m) > 1 - \beta\} \tag{3.25}$$

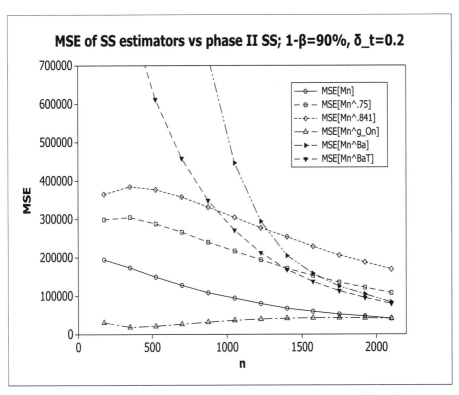

Figure 3.15 *MSE of sample size estimators of the strategies, with $\alpha = 2.5\%$ and $\delta_{0L} = 0.1$, $1 - \beta = 90\%$, $\delta_t = 0.2$.*

Bayesian SSE, provided that $T_n > 0$, is based on:

$$\hat{SP}_{2;n}^{Bas}(m) = \int_{-\infty}^{+\infty} \pi(\alpha/2, m, z)\, d\Phi_{d_n, 2/n}(z)$$

For the frequentist conservative approach of Section 3.5, when $T_n > 0$ the SP estimator is:

$$\hat{SP}_{2;n}^{\gamma}(m) = P_{d_n^{\gamma}}(T_m^* > z_{1-\alpha/2} | T_n > 0) = \Phi(d_n^{\gamma}\sqrt{m/2} - z_{1-\alpha/2}) \quad (3.26)$$

This is in accordance with two-tailed conservative RP estimation of Section 2.9.3. When $T_n \leq 0$, i.e. the pilot study provides a result in favor of the control drug, to estimate the SP is not of practical interest.

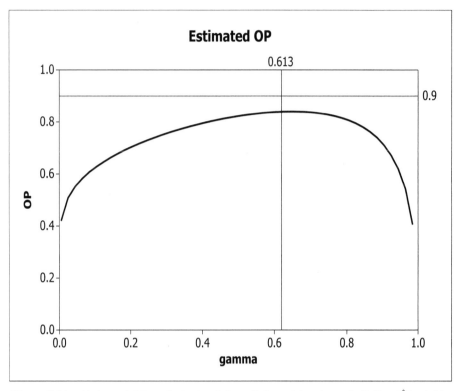

Figure 3.16   *Estimated OP on the basis of phase II data giving $d_{59} = 0.48$ (i.e. $\hat{OP}_{59}(\gamma)$), with $\alpha = 2.5\%$, $\delta_{0L} = 0.15$ and $1 - \beta = 90\%$.*

If $d_n^{\gamma} > 0$, the sample size estimator (3.25), in analogy with (3.13) and thanks to (3.26), turns out to be:

$$M_{2,n}^{\gamma} = \lfloor 2(z_{1-\alpha/2} + z_{1-\beta})^2 / (d_n^{\gamma})^2 \rfloor + 1 \tag{3.27}$$

In case $d_n^{\gamma} \leq 0$, the γ-CSSE strategy would not launch phase III.

The distribution of $M_{2,n}^{\gamma}$ in (3.27) can be computed by using (3.14) dividing α by two. So, the OP formulation in (3.17) remains valid, once again adopting $\alpha/2$. In the same way, also (3.18) and (3.19) can be used to compute the mean and MSE of $M_{2,n}^{\gamma}$. Finally, the optimal CSSE of Section 3.6 can be extended to the two-tailed setting, by just using $\alpha/2$ instead of α.

CHAPTER 4

ROBUSTNESS AND CORRECTIONS IN SAMPLE SIZE ESTIMATION

This Chapter continues to develop the arguments related to conservative sample size estimation revealed in the previous one. In fact, the problems which arise when the effect size of phase II is different from that of phase III are considered.

Indeed, broader and more heterogeneous patient populations are often pursued in phase III clinical trials as compared to those in phase II studies. This might induce larger variability and/or lower differences between means of the variables related to primary endpoints of effectiveness of different drugs. Both phenomena imply that phase III effect size δ_t is lower than the phase II one, namely δ_{II}. It should be noted that the effect the drug has is not a function of the development phase of the sponsor. Instead, there are different treatment effects for the population studied for particular phase II and phase III protocols.

In practice, when $\delta_t \neq \delta_{II}$ a structural bias arises within SSE. This difference between the effect size of the two phases in question implies that the estimation of the parameters of interest (e.g. the true effect size, the ideal sample size, the overall power) is structurally biased. Nevertheless, phase II data can be useful in estimating the sample size of phase III. The aim here is to show this usefulness.

Success Probability Estimation with Applications to Clinical Trials, First Edition.
By Daniele De Martini Copyright © 2013 John Wiley & Sons, Inc.

In this Chapter, the numerical bias of CSSE strategies is evaluated first, and their robustness is compared in different scenarios. Some techniques for correcting the bias are presented, and the changes induced on CSSE strategies are formalized. Finally, a comparison among the behavior of corrected CSSE strategies is provided.

4.1   CSSE strategies with different effect sizes in phases II and III

In this context, since phase II effect size is different from that of phase III, the formulas for CSSE should be modified. In particular, the sample size estimates, the averages and mean square errors of their values, and the OPs of their respective strategies are redefined.

Some considerations about the limits of the estimates of the quantities of interest, as the phase II sample size increases, are presented. They are derived under the condition $\delta_t < \delta_{II}$, since it is usual when the effect sizes of phase II and phase III are different. The sample size estimates are biased and they tend, for high phase II sample sizes, to a value lower than the ideal sample size M_I; the OP also tends to a value lower than the prefixed power $1 - \beta$.

The theoretical framework adopted here is analogous to that of the previous Chapter. The only difference is that phase II and phase III effect size are different: the phase II one is denoted by $\delta_{II} = (\mu_{II,1} - \mu_{II,2})/\sigma_{II}$, where $\mu_{II,i}$, $i = 1, 2$, are the true population means in phase II and σ_{II} is the common standard deviation. In other words, δ_{II} is the true effect size of phase II, not a generic one. The situation where δ_{II} is greater than the true effect size of the phase III δ_t is in study. The rate between the effect size of the two phases (i.e. δ_t/δ_{II}) is denoted by k, and k is lower than 1. In analogy with $d_n^{\bullet}$ of Section 3.2, $d_{II,n}^{\bullet}$ is a generic estimator of δ_t based on n phase II data.

The clinical relevance launch criterion is adopted in this Chapter, the difference between effect sizes does not influence equivalence among launch criteria of Section 3.3. Phase III is, therefore, launched on condition that $d_{II,n}^{\bullet} > \delta_{0L}$ (i.e. $\mathcal{L}$ iff $d_{II,n}^{\bullet} > \delta_{0L}$). In this case, the generic sample size estimator of M_I defined in analogy with (3.2) on the basis of $d_{II,n}^{\bullet}$ is denoted by $M_{II,n}^{\bullet}$, and its distribution depends, therefore, on δ_{II}, not on δ_t.

Note that $d_{II,n}^{\bullet}$ tends to δ_{II}, not δ_t. Consequently, $M_{II,n}^{\bullet}$ is not a consistent estimator of M_I, whereas it tends to $M_I k^2$.

Being $d_{II,n} = \bar{X}_{1,n} - \bar{X}_{2,n}$, the fixed-$\gamma$-conservative strategies provide $d_{II,n}^{\bullet} = d_{II,n}^{\gamma} = d_{II,n} - z_{\gamma}/\sqrt{n/2}$. According to (3.13):

$$M_{II,n}^{\gamma} = \lfloor 2(z_{1-\alpha} + z_{1-\beta})^2/(d_{II,n}^{\gamma})^2 \rfloor + 1$$

In order to apply COS, the OP is estimated by plugging $d_{II,n}$ into formula (3.17), without considering the difference between δ_{II} and δ_t.

The success probability of the Bayesian strategy in (3.22) also changes, to become:

$$\hat{SP}_n^{Bas}(m) = \int_{-\infty}^{\infty} \pi(\alpha, m, z)\phi_{d_{II,n},2/n}(z)\,dz\,,$$

where the definitions for the sample size estimators M_n^{Bas} and M_n^{BaT} remain the same.

The formulas of the average and the MSE of sample size estimators in (3.8) and (3.9) remain valid, where $M_{II,n}^{\bullet}$ replaces $M_n^{\bullet}$.

The OP in (3.12) becomes:

$$OP_n^{\bullet} = \sum_{m=2}^{M_{\max}} P_{\delta_{II}}(M_{II,n}^{\bullet} = m)SP(m) \tag{4.1}$$

This $OP_n^{\bullet}$ does not tend, as the phase II sample n increases, to the limit of consistent CSSE strategies, that is $1 - \beta$. Due to $\delta_t/\delta_{II} = k$, it tends to $SP(M_I k^2) = \pi(\alpha, M_I k^2, \delta_t)$, which is lower than $1 - \beta$ since $M_I k^2 < M_I$.

In can also be noted that the OP in (4.1) for the γ-conservative strategies introduced in Section 3.5 can be written as follows:

$$OP_n(\gamma) = \sum_{m=2}^{M_{\max}} \left[\Phi\left(\sqrt{\frac{n}{2}} \left(\frac{z_{1-\alpha} + z_{1-\beta}}{\sqrt{(m-1)/2}} - \delta_{II} \right) + z_\gamma \right) \right.$$
$$\left. -\Phi\left(\sqrt{\frac{n}{2}} \left(\frac{z_{1-\alpha} + z_{1-\beta}}{\sqrt{m/2}} - \delta_{II} \right) + z_\gamma \right) \right] \times \Phi(\delta_t \sqrt{m/2} - z_{1-\alpha}) \tag{4.2}$$

Since, remember, $\delta_{II} = \delta_t/k$, the latter formula becomes:

$$OP_n(\gamma) = \sum_{m=2}^{M_{\max}} \left[\Phi\left(\sqrt{\frac{n}{2}} \left(\frac{z_{1-\alpha} + z_{1-\beta}}{k\sqrt{(m-1)/2}} - \delta_{II} \right) + z_\gamma \right) \right.$$
$$\left. -\Phi\left(\sqrt{\frac{n}{2}} \left(\frac{z_{1-\alpha} + z_{1-\beta}}{k\sqrt{m/2}} - \delta_{II} \right) + z_\gamma \right) \right] \times \Phi(k\delta_{II} \sqrt{m/2} - z_{1-\alpha}) \tag{4.3}$$

4.2 Comparing CSSE strategies in different scenarios

A structural bias arises within SSE when $\delta_t \neq \delta_{II}$. To evaluate CSSE strategies from this perspective means to account for their robustness. To this aim, more strict launching thresholds with respect to those adopted in the previous Chapter are also considered.

Besides Scenario 1, in which the CSSE strategies have already been evaluated, three new Scenarios are introduced: Scenario 2, where δ_t is quite a bit (20%) lower than δ_{II}, and the launch threshold is set equal to the phase III effect size (i.e. $\delta_{0L} = \delta_t$); Scenario 3, where $\delta_t/\delta_{II} = 80\%$ (as in Scenario 2), and the launch threshold is set at a value somewhat lower than δ_t; Scenario 4, where δ_t is much lower than δ_{II} (50%), and the launch threshold is set as in Scenario 3.

The performances of five CSSE strategies are evaluated (viz. PWS, 3QS, 1SES, COS and BAT) by computing their OPs and the means and MSEs of their sample size estimators.

In Scenarios 2 and 4 no strategy presents robust behavior. In particular, in Scenario 2 poor performances are due to the too high launch threshold settings with respect to true effect sizes: this induces low launch probabilities, with subsequent low OPs (60% at most). Poor performances in Scenario 4 are caused by too large differences between the effect sizes of the two phases (i.e. $\delta_t << \delta_{II}$): so, sample size estimators tend to a sample size much lower than M_I (i.e. to $M_I \times 50\%^2 = M_I/4 << M_I$). The common consequence of these two Scenarios is that all strategies provide small sample size estimates, inducing low OPs.

In Scenario 3 (being this the closest to Scenario 1) all strategies are quite robust, and their OPs are higher than 70%. Nevertheless, the OPs are a bit lower than those of Scenario 1, as are the MSEs: this is a consequence of the differences between phase III and phase II effect sizes. Although COS is still the best strategy, in Scenario 3 its better performances are not as clear as in Scenario 1.

To conclude, when $\delta_t < \delta_{II}$ strict launching threshold should be avoided, whereas $\delta_{0L} \leq \delta_t/2$ is suggested. CSSE should not be applied when the effect sizes of phases II and III are far apart. When phase II effect size is moderately higher than the phase III one, CSSE can be applied and it provides useful results, particularly if COS is adopted.

4.2.1 Study design

Due to non-consistency of sample size estimators, the behavior of SSE strategies is not relevant for high values of n, either from a practical standpoint or from a theoretical one. Consequently, in order to evaluate robustness only three settings of n are considered: $n = 2M_I/3$, M_I and $4M_I/3$; $n = M_I/3$ is avoided because of the poor performances already observed in Scenario 1.

The type I error level α is set at 2.5%, as in Scenario 1, throughout the Chapter. Concerning the power, to set $1 - \beta$ equal to 80% was low even in Scenario 1. *A fortiori*, in Scenarios 2-4 where $SP(M_I k^2) < 1 - \beta$, a power choice of 80% appears to be even more penalizing. So, the power is set at $1 - \beta = 90\%$.

In Scenario 2 the settings are: $\delta_t = 0.2, 0.5, 0.8$, $k = 0.8$ (that means $\delta_t / \delta_{II} = 0.8$) and $\delta_{0L} = \delta_t$; therefore, 9 settings are considered (i.e. 3 $ns \times$ 3 δs). In Scenario 3 the launch threshold δ_{0L} is set at 0.1, with $\delta_t = 0.2, 0.5, 0.8$; then, $\delta_{0L} = 0.25$ is set, with $\delta_t = 0.5, 0.8$; as in Scenario 2, $k = 0.8$ is adopted; therefore, 15 settings (i.e. 9 + 6) are considered. In Scenario 4: $\delta_t = 0.2, 0.5, 0.8$, $k = 0.5$ and $\delta_{0L} = 0.1$, so that 9 settings are considered.

Five out of the six CSSE strategies introduced in the previous Chapter are evaluated, but only BAS is excluded due to its bad performance in Scenario 1.

4.2.2 Results

In Scenario 2 the OPs are low, ranging approximately from 27% to 63%. A discussion comparing the MSE and the average of sample size estimators is, therefore, unnecessary. These poor performances are due to too high launch threshold settings with respect to true effect sizes. This causes quite small launch probabilities, with subsequent low OPs, according to (4.3). In this Scenario the best performer is BAT, showing (on average) OPs around 60% and the lowest MSEs among sample size estimators.

In Scenario 4 the OPs are low too, ranging approximately from 38% to 55%. A fortiori the strategies are not compared. Poor performances in this Scenario are caused by too large differences between the effect sizes of the two phases, i.e. $\delta_t \ll \delta_{II}$. So, sample size estimators tend to a sample size (i.e. $M_I k^2$) much lower than the interesting one (in detail, when $k = 0.5$ the limiting sample size is $M_I / 4$). Consequently, all strategies provide small sample size estimates, inducing low OPs. The best performer is 1SES, whose OP is around 52%, and whose MSE is (on average) the lowest.

In Scenario 3 all strategies are quite robust, and their OPs are higher than 70%. Due to the difference between phase III and phase II effect sizes, the estimated sample size (i.e. $M_I k^2$) is lower than the ideal one, so that the OPs are a bit lower than those of Scenario 1. Also, the MSEs are lower than those in Scenario 1.

The performances of the CSSE strategies in 3 out of the 15 settings considered are reported in Table 4.1. Note that there is not a clear dominance of any particular strategy.

Considering the averaged behavior over all 15 settings, COS performs better than PWS, since it presents higher OP, lower MSE, and average sample size closer to M_I. COS is also better than BAT because, although the OPs of the latter is 3.3% larger than that of the former (which seems acceptable resulting 77.5%), its average sample size is closer to M_I and, in particular, it presents a dramatically lower MSE: the mean error of BAT is higher than that of COS with a factor 4.16. 3QS and 1SES perform similarly, but the former may be considered the better one: although the OP

Table 4.1   Performances of different strategies in Scenario 3, with $\delta_{0L} = 0.25$, $\delta_t = 0.5$ and $\delta_{II} = 0.625$, i.e. $k = 0.8$.

	OP, MSE and average of sample size estimators				
Overall Power - n	PWS	3QS	1SES	COS	BAT
$2M_I/3$	70.98%	75.23%	72.98%	75.19%	80.40%
M_I	72.99%	80.15%	80.67%	77.29%	80.39%
$4M_I/3$	73.68%	81.84%	83.95%	77.43%	79.77%
$MSE[M^{\bullet}_{II,n}\vert\mathcal{L}]$ - n	PWS	3QS	1SES	COS	BAT
$2M_I/3$	2716	4430	5920	939	10822
M_I	2037	3324	4614	958	5813
$4M_I/3$	1634	2454	3502	1019	3373
$E[M^{\bullet}_{II,n}\vert\mathcal{L}]$ - n	PWS	3QS	1SES	COS	BAT
$2M_I/3$	69.0	98.9	115.0	65.0	119.2
$M_I = 85$	65.7	93.0	108.6	67.7	96.5
$4M_I/3$	63.2	87.3	101.8	67.7	83.5

of 1SES is 2.0% higher, its mean error is 40% larger, and the average sample size of 3QS is 2.2 times closer to M_I than that of 1SES. 3QS provides an OP higher than that of COS (i.e. 81.7%), however COS sample size estimator performs somewhat better: the average sample size of COS is 2.0 times closer to M_I, and the mean error of 3QS is 2.2 times higher than COS. For these reasons COS is the recommended strategy even in Scenario 3.

4.3   Corrections for CSSE strategies

In the previous Section the robustness of CSSE strategies was evaluated when a structural bias was present. This bias, as well as those present in other branches of statistical theory, can nonetheless be corrected or at least reduced.

To this aim, a different type I error α can be adopted (e.g. 0.5% instead of 2.5%), or a different power $1 - \beta$ can be set (e.g. 95% instead of 90%). Moreover, both corrections can be applied simultaneously. This different type I error level would be, nonetheless, adopted just to estimate phase III sample size, not to evaluate the significance of phase III outcomes.

A more intuitive technique of bias reduction consists in focusing on the rate between the effect sizes of the two phases, that is on $k = \delta_t/\delta_{II}$. In practice, by speculating on the structural bias, a value for k is given, namely k_c where

c stands for *correction*. Then, k_c is applied to the estimate of phase III effect size based on the (biased) phase II data to reduce its implicit bias. For example, being $d_{II,n}^{\gamma}$ the γ-conservative estimate of δ_t, then its k_c-corrected estimate is $d_{II,n}^{\gamma} \times k_c$.

From a mathematical perspective, the correction techniques based on modifying the type I error or/and the power are connected to that based on the postulated k, i.e. k_c.

The correction based on k_c can be applied to CSSE strategies, and their related formulas for SSE are presented, together with the derivation of the OP.

4.3.1 Corrections and their equivalence

Correcting error levels. In the presence of a structural bias, modification of the type I error and/or the power is sometimes suggested. In practice an α^* (usually lower than α) or/and an $1 - \beta^*$ (usually higher than the nominal power) are set in order just to estimate the sample size: they are neither used to evaluate significance of phase III outcomes nor to mean that a certain power is desired. In other words α^* and $1 - \beta^*$ are not the targeted significance level and the targeted power, they merely influence sample size estimators.

For example, by adopting $1 - \beta^*$ instead of $1 - \beta$ the γ-conservative sample size estimator M_n^{γ} in (3.13) becomes:

$$M_{II,n}^{\gamma*} = \lfloor 2(z_{1-\alpha} + z_{1-\beta^*})^2/(d_{II,n}^{\gamma})^2 \rfloor + 1$$

Note also that launch criteria are not modified conceptually, whereas the new maximum sample size is $M_{max}^* = \lfloor 2(z_{1-\alpha} + z_{1-\beta^*})^2/(\delta_{0L})^2 \rfloor + 1$.

For further details on these kind of corrections see Wang et al. (2006). Nevertheless, their conclusions are based on the computation of the average of sample size estimators only, not on MSE and OP evaluations (see Table 4 in their work).

Postulating the correction for the effect size. This technique concerns a correction to be applied directly on the effect size estimator $d_{II,n}^{\bullet}$, and it has been presented in De Martini (2011c).

The proposed approach stems from two observations: on the one hand, CSSE aims at studying the performances of $M_{II,n}^{\bullet}$ based on $d_{II,n}^{\bullet}$, which, in Scenarios 2-4, is a biased (and not consistent) estimator of δ_t; on the other hand, the structural bias can be modeled through the relation $k = \delta_t/\delta_{II}$.

Hence, to improve CSSE performances one can naturally and intuitively speculate first about k. Being k_c the postulated correction, the sample size estimator $M_n^{\bullet}$ in (3.2) can be directly modified by using $d_{II,n}^{\bullet} \times k_c$ instead of $d_{II,n}^{\bullet}$ only, obtaining a sample size estimator denoted by $_cM_{II,n}^{\bullet}$. For example, in the frequentist framework

(3.4) becomes:

$$_{c}M^{\bullet}_{II,n} = \lfloor 2(z_{1-\alpha} + z_{1-\beta})^2/(d^{\bullet}_{II,n} \times k_c)^2 \rfloor + 1$$

The maximum sample size, consequently, changes, and the new one is:

$$_{c}M_{\max} = \lfloor 2(z_{1-\alpha} + z_{1-\beta})^2/(\delta_{0L} \times k_c)^2 \rfloor + 1 \qquad (4.4)$$

Note that if the postulated correction k_c is right (i.e. $k_c = \delta_t/\delta_t$), then CSSE strategies are consistent: $_{c}M^{\bullet}_{II,n}$ tends to M_I. Nevertheless, in this circumstance we are still not in Scenario 1: although the mean of $_{c}d_{II,n}$ is actually δ_t, its variance is $2k_c^2/n$, which is different from that of $d_{II,n}$ in Scenario 1, which was $2/n$ (as explained in Section 1.1).

Equivalence of corrections. When $M^{\bullet}_{II,n}$ is a γ-conservative estimator belonging to the family introduced in Section 3.5, the two corrections above are equivalent.

Indeed, both approaches aim to correct $M^{\gamma}_{II,n} = \lfloor 2(z_{1-\alpha} + z_{1-\beta})^2/(d^{\gamma}_{II,n})^2 \rfloor + 1$ in order to make the latter closer to M_I. Corrections can be made to the numerator (as α^* and β^* do) or to the denominator (as k_c does). For each correction on the numerator there exists an equivalent correction for the denominator. For example, for every $\beta^* < \beta$ there exists $k_c < 1$ such that $z_{1-\alpha} + z_{1-\beta^*} = (z_{1-\alpha} + z_{1-\beta})/k_c$.

Finally, note that the launch probability is not modified by either kind of corrections. Indeed, $d^{\bullet}_{II,n}$ remains the same, as well as $P_{\delta_{II}}(\mathcal{L}) = P_{\delta_{II}}(d^{\bullet}_{II,n} > \delta_{0L})$; $M^{\bullet}_{II,n}$ alone is modified.

4.3.2 Corrected CSSE strategies

Although the corrections are equivalent on $M^{\gamma}_{II,n}$ only, the one based on the direct postulated correction k_c is applied to CSSE strategies because it is considered more intuitive and easy to apply.

Corrected frequentist conservative strategies (viz. PWS, 1SES, 3QS). The corrected γ-conservative estimator of δ_t is obtained by multiplying the conservative effect size estimator based on phase II data for the correction k_c. Formally, we have: $_{c}d^{\gamma}_{II,n} = (d_{II,n} - z_{\gamma}/\sqrt{n/2}) \times k_c$. Then, the corrected fixed-γ CSSE strategy provides:

$$_{c}M^{\gamma}_{II,n} = \lfloor 2(z_{1-\alpha} + z_{1-\beta})^2/(_{c}d^{\gamma}_{II,n})^2 \rfloor + 1$$

Corrected COS. Consider first the corrected version of the estimated OP. Following from (4.3), where k_c and $d_{II,n}$ substituted k and δ_{II} into that part of the formula regarding the distribution of the sample size estimator, and $k_c \times d_{II,n}$ substituted $k \times \delta_{II}$ into that of the SP:

$$
{}_c\hat{OP}_n(\gamma) = \sum_{m=2}^{{}_cM_{\max}} \left[\Phi\left(\sqrt{\frac{n}{2}} \left(\frac{z_{1-\alpha} + z_{1-\beta}}{k_c\sqrt{(m-1)/2}} - d_{II,n} \right) + z_\gamma \right) \right.
$$

$$
\left. - \Phi\left(\sqrt{\frac{n}{2}} \left(\frac{z_{1-\alpha} + z_{1-\beta}}{k_c\sqrt{m/2}} - d_{II,n} \right) + z_\gamma \right) \right] \times \Phi(k_c d_{II,n}\sqrt{m/2} - z_{1-\alpha}) \quad (4.5)
$$

Now, denote by g_n^O the argument of the constrained maximum of (4.5), according to (3.21). Then, make use of ${}_c d_{II,n}^{g_n^O} = (d_{II,n} - z_{g_n^O}/\sqrt{n/2}) \times k_c$ to define the sample size estimator ${}_c M_{II,n}^{g_n^O}$, i.e. the corrected estimator of the COS, by plugging it into (3.13) in place of d_n^γ.

Corrected BAS and BAT. In order to correct Bayesian strategies, the postulated k_c is applied to the estimated success probability estimator in (3.22), which becomes:

$$
{}_c\hat{SP}_n^{Bas}(m) = \int_{-\infty}^{\infty} \pi(\alpha, m, z \times k_c)\phi_{d_{II,n}, 2/n}(z)\, dz
$$

According to (3.2), the classical estimated sample size so obtained is, therefore, ${}_c M_{II,n}^{Bas} = \min\{m \mid {}_c\hat{SP}_n^{Bas}(m) > 1 - \beta\}$. As a consequence of (4.4), the truncated Bayesian strategy gives ${}_c M_{II,n}^{BaT} = \min\{{}_c M_{II,n}^{Bas}, {}_c M_{\max}\}$.

4.4   A comparison among corrected CSSE strategies

In light of the poor performances shown by CSSE in Scenarios 2 and 4, only Scenario 3 is studied. The considered rate between different effect sizes is $\delta_t/\delta_{II} = 80\%$, and the launch threshold is set at a value somewhat lower than δ_t. Three possible corrections are evaluated: the right one, the one obtained with a 10% increase from the right one and the one with a 10% decrease.

With a higher than necessary correction, the OPs of all strategies result higher than the prefixed power, but also the mean error and the bias of sample size estimates increase a lot with respect to Scenario 3 without corrections. This is caused by too high sample size estimates provided by this excessive correction. It would therefore be preferable to avoid higher than necessary corrections.

The smaller than necessary correction works well: the slight increase in MSEs with respect to the uncorrected performances in Scenario 3 is counter balanced by the good improvements in OPs for all strategies, once again with respect to Scenario 3 without corrections. COS turns out to be the best performer.

With the right correction (i.e. $k_c = k$) all strategies are consistent, as phase II sample size tends to ∞: their OPs tend to the prefixed power $1 - \beta$ and their MSEs tend to zero. Here again COS is recommended, and this was to be expected since postulating the right correction makes CSSE close to that in Scenario 1.

It is worth noting that the OPs provided by all corrected strategies are, in the latter favorable circumstance, a little higher (and closer to $1 - \beta$) than those computed in Scenario 1 (see Figure 4.1); moreover, the MSEs are comparable to those in Scenario 1 (see Figure 4.2). These behaviors are due to the higher launch probabilities with respect to Scenario 1 (due to $\delta_{II} > \delta_t$), and to the quite close SSE performances.

It follows that the structural bias $\delta_{II} > \delta_t$ can be exploited for improving CSSE, should the right correction be applied.

Even in the presence of structural bias it is maintained that the operating conditions for CSSE are: the launch threshold should be set lower than one half the true phase III effect size; the pilot sample should be around the ideal one (i.e. $n \geq 2M_I/3$); a power of 90% should be adopted.

4.4.1   Study design

Scenario 3 only is examined, with $\delta_{0L} = 0.1$, $\delta_t = 0.2, 0.5, 0.8$, $k = \delta_t/\delta_{II} = 0.8$, and with $n = 2M_I/3$, M_I and $4M_I/3$.

As regards k_c, there are three postulated corrections: a smaller than necessary one, i.e. $k_c = 0.9$, the right one, i.e. $k_c = 0.8$, and a higher than necessary one, i.e. $k_c = 0.7$. So, 27 settings are evaluated (3 ns $\times$ 3 δ_3s $\times$ 3 k_cs).

Since our CSSE strategies are consistent when $k_c = 0.8$, their asymptotic behavior is also evaluated, with n up to $4M_I$, for the three δ_ts. Once again, the OPs of CSSE strategies, and the MSEs and averages of their sample size estimators are taken into account.

Remark 4.1. *Simple algebra provides that when $k_c < 1$ both the average and the standard deviation of $_cM^\gamma_{II,n}$ increase $1/k_c$ times with respect to those of $M^\gamma_{II,n}$. As a consequence, $MSE[_cM^\gamma_{II,n}]$ is often higher than $MSE[M^\gamma_{II,n}]$. An analogous behavior for the corrected COS and BAT is expected.*

4.4.2   Results

When a correction $k_c < 1$ is applied the OPs of all strategies improve. Moreover, according to Remark 4.1 above, MSEs and averages of sample size estimators increase, as seen in Table 4.2. The bias of $_cM^\gamma_{II,n}$ augments too in all circumstances but one (i.e. for PWS with $k_c = 0.9$).

With the higher than necessary correction of $k_c = 0.7$, the OPs of all strategies result higher than 90%, going, on average, from 92.3% (PWS) to 95.1% (BAT) (COS

Table 4.2 Performances of corrected strategies in Scenario 3, where $\delta_t/\delta_{II} = k = 0.8$, with $\delta_{0L} = 0.1$ and $\delta_t = 0.5$.

Overall Power	n	OP, MSE and average of sample size estimators				
		PWS	3QS	1SES	COS	BAT
	$2M_I/3$	79.49%	87.54%	88.97%	84.66%	87.17%
$k_c = 0.9$	M_I	80.51%	88.78%	91.50%	84.09%	86.54%
	$4M_I/3$	80.97%	88.85%	91.80%	83.71%	85.94%
	$2M_I/3$	85.81%	91.54%	91.90%	89.53%	91.48%
$k_c = 0.8$	M_I	87.09%	93.13%	94.79%	89.68%	91.48%
	$4M_I/3$	87.71%	93.48%	95.40%	89.73%	91.32%
	$2M_I/3$	91.48%	94.71%	94.08%	93.81%	95.10%
$k_c = 0.7$	M_I	92.79%	96.44%	97.13%	94.39%	95.48%
	$4M_I/3$	93.42%	96.91%	97.89%	94.65%	95.58%
$MSE[_cM^\bullet_{II,n}|\mathcal{L}]$	n	PWS	3QS	1SES	COS	BAT
	$2M_I/3$	19280	72276	124432	6780	356741
$k_c = 0.9$	M_I	5216	26411	53015	5451	91625
	$4M_I/3$	2189	11746	25536	3847	22324
	$2M_I/3$	32249	121648	208530	13047	583438
$k_c = 0.8$	M_I	8861	45782	90724	10315	151353
	$4M_I/3$	3658	21134	44867	7164	37806
	$2M_I/3$	58518	217829	371002	26981	1014780
$k_c = 0.7$	M_I	17304	84775	164929	21440	266519
	$4M_I/3$	7889	40968	83939	15181	69011
$E[_cM^\bullet_{II,n}|\mathcal{L}]$	n	PWS	3QS	1SES	COS	BAT
	$2M_I/3$	100.3	179.8	238.0	114.0	287.0
$k_c = 0.9$	$M_I = 85$	85.0	137.4	178.2	103.6	156.9
	$4M_I/3$	78.8	116.9	145.9	93.5	112.3
	$2M_I/3$	126.8	227.4	301.1	144.4	364.3
$k_c = 0.8$	$M_I = 85$	107.5	173.8	225.4	131.2	198.5
	$4M_I/3$	99.5	147.9	184.6	118.4	142.0
	$2M_I/3$	165.5	296.8	393.1	188.7	475.7
$k_c = 0.7$	$M_I = 85$	140.3	226.8	294.2	171.5	259.1
	$4M_I/3$	129.9	193.0	240.9	154.7	185.3

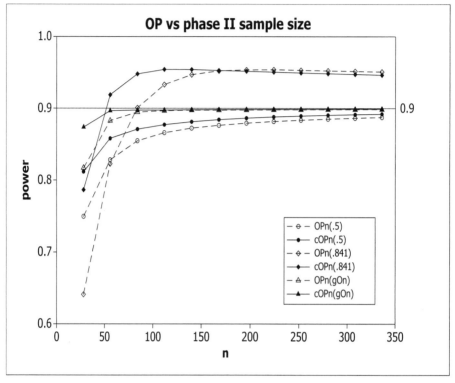

Figure 4.1   *Overall Powers of PWS, 1SES and COS in Scenario 3 (where $\delta_t/\delta_{II} = k = 0.8$), with the right correction $k_c = 0.8$ and in Scenario 1, with $\alpha = 2.5\%$, $1 - \beta = 90\%$, $\delta_t = 0.5$ and $\delta_{0L} = 0.1$.*

provided 94.0%). Nevertheless, the $MSE^{1/2}$ increases, on average, from 2.14 times with PWS to 2.46 times with COS, with respect to those obtained without correction. Also, the averages of sample size estimators are much higher than M_I. These performances are caused by too high sample size estimates provided by this excessive correction. As regards detailed results, the $MSE^{1/2}$ of COS is once again the lowest: the enlargements of the other strategies go from 12% of PWS to 331% of BAT.

With $k_c = 0.9$ OPs improve, on average over the 9 settings, from 4% with 1SES to 6.8% with PWS, but they are still lower than 90% (from 80.1% of PWS to 88.5% of 1SES). The $MSE^{1/2}$ of corrected strategies increases, on average, with respect to the uncorrected ones, from 16% with PWS (i.e. $MSE^{1/2}$ of corrected PWS is 1.16 times higher than that of PWS without any correction) to 30% of 1SES. Hence, this correction works well because the small increase in MSEs is counter balanced by the good improvements in OPs. In particular, the OP of COS increases 6.1%, on average, becoming 83.7% (3QS, 87.1%). The corrected COS provides the second best improvement in OP and the second smallest increase in $MSE^{1/2}$ (19%). Moreover, the $MSE^{1/2}$ of COS is still the lowest: those of PWS, 3QS, 1SES and BAT are, on average, 1.28, 2.53, 3.53 and 5.04 times higher, respectively. Since COS was the best performer in the uncorrected Scenario 3, it remains the recommended strategy even with a smaller than necessary correction.

With the right correction $k_c = 0.8$ all strategies converge, as n tends to ∞: their OPs tend to 90% and their MSEs tend to zero (see Figures 4.1 and 4.2). It should also be noted that when $2M_I \leq n \leq 4M_I/3$, all strategies provide OPs closer to 90% than those obtained with $k_c = 0.9$. Furthermore, considering the latter pilot sample sizes, COS converges faster. Indeed, the strategy with averaged OP (over the usual 9 settings) closest to 90% is COS (89.4%), where the highest differences are provided by 1SES (91.8%). The $MSE^{1/2}$ increases, as expected, from 51% of PWS to 74% of 1SES, with respect to that provided by the strategies without correction. Also, the MSE of COS is the lowest: the enlargements in $MSE^{1/2}$ go from 21% of PWS to 4.75 times (i.e. 375%) of BAT. Once again COS is recommended, and this was to be expected, since postulating the right correction makes sample size estimations quite close to those in Scenario 1.

In conclusion, it is worth noting that the OPs provided by all corrected strategies are a little higher (and closer to 90%) than the respective ones computed in Scenario 1 where a correction was not needed (see Figure 4.1; see also De Martini, 2011b). When the right correction is applied (i.e. $k_c = 0.8$) the MSEs are comparable to, and often lower than, those in Scenario 1 (see Figure 4.2). This means that applying the right correction, the OPs are higher and the MSEe are often lower than those in Scenario 1. In other words, having a structural bias and correcting it properly can, paradoxically, improve CSSE performances with respect to those of Scenario 1 where a correction is not needed. This unexpected result is due to higher launch probabilities with respect to those in Scenario 1 (due to $\delta_{II} > \delta_t$), and to quite close behaviors of sample size estimators.

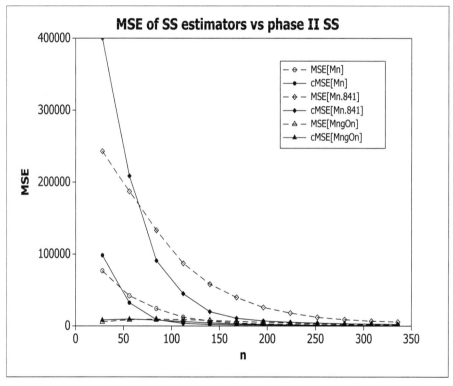

Figure 4.2   *MSEs of the sample size estimators of PWS, 1SES and COS in Scenario 3 (where $\delta_t/\delta_{II} = k = 0.8$), with the right correction $k_c = 0.8$ and in Scenario 1, with $\alpha = 2.5\%$, $1 - \beta = 90\%$, $\delta_t = 0.5$ and $\delta_{0L} = 0.1$.*

PART II

SUCCESS PROBABILITY ESTIMATION FOR SOME WIDELY USED STATISTICAL TESTS

In the second part of the book the techniques for SP estimation are studied in depth. Applications to both RP estimation, as in Chapter 2, and to CSSE, as in Chapters 3 and 4 are provided. The language adopted is more formal (in the mathematical-statistical sense) than that of Part I.

In Chapter 5 a general parametric setting for the distribution of the test statistic, which is based on two independent samples from different distributions, is considered. A general technique for SP estimation is provided. Then, RP estimation, together with RP-testing, and CSSE are derived for a wide class of parametric tests.

In the remaining Chapters 6-9 some statistical tests for comparing the outcomes of two groups, as if the two-arm parallel design were adopted, are taken into account. For these tests RP estimation and CSSE are studied in depth, illustrated and exemplified.

Success Probability Estimation with Applications to Clinical Trials, First Edition.
By Daniele De Martini Copyright © 2013 John Wiley & Sons, Inc.

Following the SP estimation technique revealed in Chapter 5, some parametric situations are studied in Chapters 6-8. In Chapter 6 the tests to compare two means with unknown variances (both with equal or unequal variances) are considered, which refer to the Student's t distribution. Then, the test to compare two proportions and the one to compare two survival rates over time (i.e. two survival curves) are discussed together in Chapter 7, since they both refer to the Gaussian distribution. Finally, the test to compare two C-categorical variables (i.e. two multinomial distributions) and the one to compare two proportions among some different strata, both referring to the χ^2 distribution, are presented in Chapter 8.

In Chapter 9 a nonparametric framework, where the distributions of the variables of interest are unknown, is considered. A general nonparametric technique for SP estimation is provided, which can be applied to many nonparametric tests. In particular, focus is placed on RP estimation and CSSE of the well known Wilcoxon rank-sum test.

CHAPTER 5

GENERAL PARAMETRIC SP ESTIMATION

In this Chapter, SP estimation is extended to a general parametric model. Firstly, this model is presented, which considers families of distributions based on a single non-centrality parameter. Then, it is shown that the power function of the test depends on the noncentrality parameter, whose estimation is the basis for performing SP estimation. Consequently, RP estimation and RP-testing are presented in the general context of the model, as well as conservative sample size estimation. Finally, some examples of applications are given, introducing those more related to clinical trials that will be extensively illustrated in the following Chapters.

5.1 The parametric model

The parametric model for comparing some features of two distributions, i.e. for testing differences among the latter, is introduced here and a general theoretical framework is adopted.

Let us define F_1 as the generic distribution of the variable of interest of the population under the new treatment and F_2 as that of the control population. The couple (F_1, F_2)

belongs to a family of couples of distributions $\mathcal{F}$ over a space $S \subset R \times R$. The latter family is divided into two parts: $\mathcal{F}_0$, containing the couples representing an ineffective new treatment, and its complement $\mathcal{F}\backslash\mathcal{F}_0$.

Being $_tF_1$ and $_tF_2$ the true, unknown, distributions the null hypothesis is $H_0 :$ $(_tF_1, _tF_2) \in \mathcal{F}_0$ and the alternative hypothesis of effectiveness of the new drug is $H_1 : (_tF_1, _tF_2) \in \mathcal{F}\backslash\mathcal{F}_0$.

The random variables $X_{1,1}, \ldots, X_{1,m_1}$ are assumed to be independent and identically distributed, with distribution $_tF_1$. Analogously, $X_{2,1}, \ldots, X_{2,m_2}$ represent a sample from $_tF_2$. Moreover $m = (m_1, m_2)$ is set and the whole sample from both populations is $\mathbf{X_m} = \{X_{1,1}, \ldots, X_{1,m_1}; X_{2,1}, \ldots, X_{2,m_2}\}$.

The test statistic is $T_m = \mathcal{T}(\mathbf{X_m}) \in R$ and it has a parametric continuous distribution $G_{m, _t\lambda_m}$, where $_t\lambda_m \in R$ is the true parameter of noncentrality. This $_t\lambda_m$ can usually be written as a function of the parameters of $_tF_1$ and $_tF_2$ and of m. To fix the idea, reference is made to the situation studied in the first part of the book, that is the comparison of the means of two normal distributions with known equal variances σ^2, where $_t\lambda_m = \sqrt{m_1m_2/(m_1 + m_2)}(\mu_1 - \mu_2)/\sigma$. In detail, under the conditions of $m_1 = m_2$ and of $\sigma = 1$ adopted in previous chapters, $_t\lambda_m$ turns out to be $\delta_t\sqrt{m_1/2}$.

Then, it is assumed that $\sup_{H_0}\{_t\lambda_m\} = \lambda_0$ and that G_{m,λ_0} is known. Being α the type I error probability, and considering the one-tailed test, $t_{m,1-\alpha} = G_{m,\lambda_0}^{-1}(1 - \alpha)$ is the critical value of the following statistical test:

$$\psi_\alpha(T_m) = \begin{cases} 1 & \text{if} \quad T_m > t_{m,1-\alpha} \\ 0 & \text{if} \quad T_m \leq t_{m,1-\alpha} \end{cases} \tag{5.1}$$

The p-value is the type I error that should have been defined in order to find the test statistic T_m on the boundary of the rejection region, i.e. the p-value is such that $T_m = t_{m,1-\text{p-value}}$. In formulas we have:

$$\text{p-value} = 1 - G_{m,\lambda_0}(T_m) \tag{5.2}$$

A classical study of statistical hypotheses testing can be found in Lehmann and Romano (2005).

5.2 Power, SP and noncentrality parameter estimation

Let λ_m be the generic noncentrality parameter, depending on the generic distributions F_1 and F_2. The power function of the test is:

$$\pi(\alpha, \lambda_m) = P_{\lambda_m}(T_m > t_{m,1-\alpha}) = 1 - G_{m,\lambda_m}(t_{m,1-\alpha}) \tag{5.3}$$

Note that, since m is embedded in λ_m, the power function π depends only implicitly on m. Hence, through the definition (5.3) and $_t\lambda_m$ the success probability is:

$$SP = P_{t\lambda_m}(T_m > t_{m,1-\alpha}) = \pi(\alpha, {}_t\lambda_m) \tag{5.4}$$

This is in accordance with (1.11) where $_t\lambda_m = \delta_t\sqrt{m_1/2}$.

Exact confidence intervals for $_t\lambda_m$ can be computed under the condition of stochastic increasing ordering of the family of distributions G_{m,λ_m}. This condition consists in fulfilling:

$$G_{m,\lambda'_m}(x) > G_{m,\lambda''_m}(x) \quad \forall x \in R \quad \text{if} \quad \lambda'_m < \lambda''_m \tag{5.5}$$

A γ-lower bound for the noncentrality parameter (namely ℓ_m^γ) is obtained by solving the following nonlinear equation in v, which involves the test statistic T_m and the noncentral distribution $G_{m,{}_t\lambda_m}$:

$$G_{m,v}(T_m) = \gamma \tag{5.6}$$

This nonlinear equation can be solved numerically, for example, through the bisection method, and the resulting solution v is ℓ_m^γ. Then the latter quantity is actually a lower bound for $_t\lambda_m$:

$$P_{({}_tF_1, {}_tF_2)}(\ell_m^\gamma \le {}_t\lambda_m) = \gamma$$

5.3   RP estimation and testing

Assume now that two samples of size n_1 and n_2 have been drawn from $_tF_1$ and $_tF_2$, respectively ($n = (n_1, n_2)$). According to Section 2.1, the SP in (5.4) evaluated when $m = n$ assumes the meaning of Reproducibility Probability - RP, i.e. $RP = \pi(\alpha, {}_t\lambda_n)$. From (5.6) the lower bound for the noncentrality parameter (i.e. ℓ_n^γ) can, therefore, be computed.

A γ lower bound for the RP can be obtained by plugging ℓ_n^γ into the power function (5.3), obtaining:

$$\pi(\alpha, \ell_n^\gamma) = \hat{RP}_\alpha^\gamma \tag{5.7}$$

fulfilling:

$$P(\hat{RP}_\alpha^\gamma \le RP) = \gamma$$

A pointwise estimator of the RP is obtained with $\gamma = 1/2$: it is simply denoted by $\hat{RP}_\alpha$, instead of $\hat{RP}_\alpha^{1/2}$. The possibility of referring to the estimates given by $\hat{RP}_\alpha$ to test statistical hypotheses holds also in this general parametric framework

(De Martini, 2008), and so:

$$\psi_\alpha(T_m) = \begin{cases} 1 & \text{if } \hat{R}P_\alpha > 1/2 \\ 0 & \text{if } \hat{R}P_\alpha \le 1/2 \end{cases} \tag{5.8}$$

Finally, stability evaluations can be applied in this general context, according to the definitions of Sections 2.4, 2.5 and 2.6. Lower bounds for RP (i.e. $\hat{R}P_\alpha^\gamma$) can be adopted. In particular, γ-stability is achieved when $\hat{R}P_\alpha^\gamma > 1/2$.

5.4 Sample size estimation

First, the notation which recalls that the SP is a function of the sample size is adopted and so the SP in (5.4) is denoted by $SP(m)$. Hence, given the power $1 - \beta$, the ideal sample size is:

$$M_I = \min\{m : SP(m) > 1 - \beta\} = \min\{m : 1 - G_{m, t\lambda_m}(t_{m,1-\alpha}) > 1 - \beta\} \tag{5.9}$$

When a pilot data is available the true noncentrality parameter $_t\lambda_m$, and consequently also M_I, can be estimated. Actually, in order to estimate M_I conservatively, a lower bound for $_t\lambda_m$ is needed.

Here, the problem is that the size of the sample is embedded in the estimator of the noncentrality parameter. In detail, when a sample of size n is available $_t\lambda_n$ can be estimated through ℓ_n^γ, whereas $_t\lambda_m$ cannot. Nevertheless, a lower bound for the latter can usually be obtained from ℓ_n^γ through simple algebra on m and n. In practice, often:

$$\ell_{m,n}^\gamma = \ell_n^\gamma \frac{l(m)}{l(n)} \tag{5.10}$$

where $l()$ assumes the role of *link* function.

For example, when the means of two normal distributions with known equal variances are compared $\ell_n^\gamma = \sqrt{n_1 n_2/(n_1 + n_2)}(\bar{X}_{1,n_1} - \bar{X}_{2,n_2})/\sigma - z_\gamma$ and $l(u_1, u_2) = \sqrt{u_1 u_2/(u_1 + u_2)}$.

The adoption of $\ell_{m,n}^\gamma$ in (5.10) brings to the possibility of estimating $SP(m)$ conservatively:

$$\hat{S}P_n^\gamma(m) = 1 - G_{m, \ell_{m,n}^\gamma}(t_{m,1-\alpha}) \tag{5.11}$$

and then to estimate M_I according to (3.13), that is:

$$M_n^\gamma = \min\{m : 1 - G_{m, \ell_{m,n}^\gamma}(t_{m,1-\alpha}) > 1 - \beta\} \tag{5.12}$$

Regarding the three launching criteria of Section 3.3, they are still mathematically equivalent. Nevertheless, in some circumstances the one based on clinical relevance is not recommended because the effect size is either ambiguous, or it is difficult to evaluate its amplitude (as will be shown later). For these reasons, adopting either the one based on statistical significance of phase II data, or that based on the maximum sample size is suggested.

As a consequence of the launching condition the OP of γ-CSSE strategies, in analogy with Section 3.5, results:

$$OP_n(\gamma) = \sum_{m=2}^{M_{\max}} (1 - G_{m,{}_t\lambda_m}(t_{m,1-\alpha}))P(M_n^\gamma = m) \tag{5.13}$$

Note that the last factor of the summands (i.e. $P(M_n^\gamma = m)$) is not explicitly affected by the conditioning on launch, according to (3.17). The launching condition is, indeed, embedded in the limit of $M_{\max}$ thanks to the equivalence of launching criteria.

The OP in (5.13) can be estimated in order to then apply COS, in analogy with Section 3.6. Nevertheless, it will be shown that in specific cases some technical difficulties arise.

In order to apply Bayesian CSSE, a prior distribution for ${}_t\lambda_m$ may be specified, but the problem of integrating over that prior to obtain the Bayesian posterior distribution arises. A simpler approach consists in adopting the *fiducial distribution* for ${}_t\lambda_m$ instead of the posterior, as suggested by Fay et al. (2007). In this way, the Bayesian SP estimator analogous to that in (3.23) is derived by exploiting (5.11):

$$\hat{SP}_n^{Bas}(m) = \int_0^1 \hat{SP}_n^\gamma(m)d\gamma = 1 - \int_0^1 G_{m,\ell_{m,n}^\gamma}(t_{m,1-\alpha})d\gamma$$

and the Bayesian sample size estimators M_n^{Bas} and M_n^{BaT} can be obtained.

Appropriated corrections to sample size estimators based on phase II data can be applied. The corrections are analogous to those discussed in Section 4.3, which consisted in modifying either error levels or, directly, the effect size estimators. The latter corrections will be discussed for some of the statistical tests presented in the next Section.

5.5   Statistical tests included in the model

The model introduced in Section 5.1, under which RP-testing holds and conservative sample size estimation can be performed, is very general. Here, it is shown that many practical and very often encountered testing situations are included in the model, so that for these tests RP-testing and CSSE can be applied.

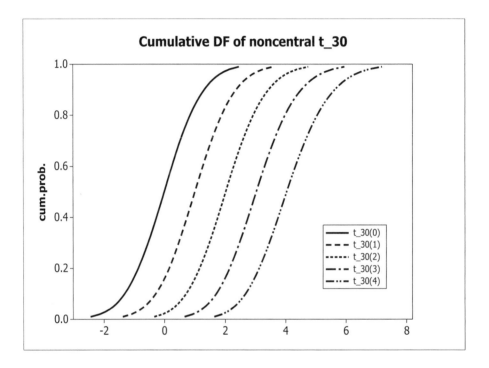

Figure 5.1   *Stochastic ordering of t distributions, with 30 dfs and noncentrality parameter equal to* $= 0, 1, 2, 3, 4$.

As it concerns the family of distributions G_{m,λ_m}, it has to fulfill the stochastic ordering in (5.5). This requirement can be viewed as a mild condition, indeed many widely applied families of distribution are included. For example, G_{m,λ_m} can be: the Gaussian distribution with mean λ_m and unitary variance (i.e. $\Phi_{(\lambda_m,1)}$); the noncentral t with noncentrality parameter λ_m (i.e. $\tau_{f(m),\lambda_m}$, where $f(m)$ represents the number of *Degrees of Freedom* - dfs); the noncentral χ^2, that is χ^2_{C,λ_m} (where C represents the number of dfs); the noncentral Fisher's F, F_{C_1,C_2,λ_m} (C_1, C_2 dfs). Other families of distributions are also included (e.g. the Gamma distribution), but the test statistic T_m often has a distribution belonging to one of the four families above (statistical distributions can be found, for example, in Forbes et al., 2011).

In order to better understand what stochastic ordering (5.5) means, Figures 5.1 and 5.2 show the stochastic increasing ordering of t and χ^2 distributions (with 30 and 3 dfs respectively). Varying the noncentrality parameter, t distributions maintain the same shape (as Gaussian distributions do), whereas χ^2 distributions do not (as F distributions). It can be noted that in both cases condition (5.5) is fulfilled.

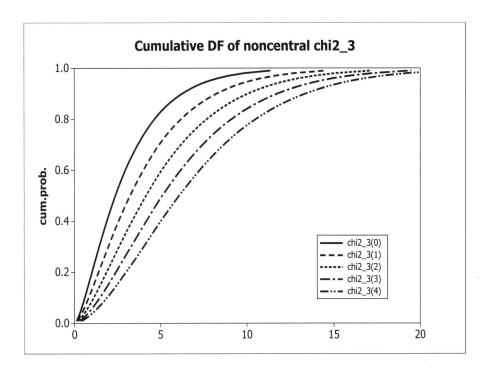

Figure 5.2 *Stochastic ordering of χ^2 distributions, with 3 dfs and noncentrality parameter equal to = 0, 1, 2, 3, 4.*

With regard to two-tailed tests, RP estimation can be reduced to that of the one-tailed setting, in analogy with Section 2.9. In particular, remember that $\hat{RP}_{2;\alpha} = \hat{RP}_{\alpha/2}$, and that the tail where the RP is estimated is that where the test statistic falls. Lower bounds for RP follows. In sample size estimation too, $\alpha/2$ should be adopted in place of α. As a consequence, two-sided alternative situations can be faced, whether the test is one- or two-tailed.

When clinical superiority and clinical non-inferiority hypotheses are under testing, the threshold δ_0 of clinical relevance can be embedded in the test statistic T_m, according to test statistic definitions in Section 1.8.

Many asymptotic solutions of statistical testing refer to the Gaussian distribution, for example the widely applied tests on proportions (see Chapter 7). Then, many others refer to the t distribution, for example, the tests on regression parameters in a linear model (see Searle, 1971) or simply tests on means comparison with unknown variances (see Chapter 6). χ^2 distribution are often used too, for example in presence of contingency tables (see Chapter 8), or survival analysis, or generalized linear models (see Agresti, 2002, Collett, 2003, McCullagh and Nelder, 1989, respectively). Also, analysis of variance tests refer to the F distribution (see Scheffé, 1999). Consequently, RP-testing and CSSE can be applied in a very large number of these testing situations through the techniques here shown.

In the following Chapters, SP estimation for some parametric tests that are often applied in clinical research will be studied in detail. These tests are included in the general model above. In particular, statistical tests for comparing the outcomes of two groups will be taken into consideration, as if a two-arm parallel design were adopted. Some statistical tests whose test statistics follow: the Gaussian family of distributions, the t, the χ^2 families, will be considered.

CHAPTER 6

SP ESTIMATION FOR STUDENT'S T STATISTICAL TESTS

This Chapter considers some tests whose test statistic is distributed as a Student's t. It would seem more natural to present this Chapter after those concerning Gaussian and χ^2 distributions, since the Student's t, as a distribution, is derived from the two distributions above. Nevertheless, it is preferable to first extend the framework considered in the first part of the book (i.e. comparison of two means) to the analogous one where the standard deviations of the two groups are unknown.

Thus, SP estimation is shown here for the tests for comparing the means of two groups whose outcomes have Gaussian distributions with unknown variances, under the conditions of equal and unequal variances. In both cases the test statistic is distributed as a Student's t. Two tests will therefore be considered, where G_{m,λ_m} is a t distribution with a number of dfs depending on m (i.e. $f(m)$) and noncentrality parameter λ_m, that is, $G_{m,\lambda_m} = \tau_{f(m),\lambda_m}$.

Success Probability Estimation with Applications to Clinical Trials, First Edition.
By Daniele De Martini Copyright © 2013 John Wiley & Sons, Inc.

6.1   Test for two means - equal variances

The true distribution $_tF_1$ of the variable of interest for the population treated with the new drug is assumed to be the Gaussian $N(\mu_1, \sigma^2)$, whereas that of the control population is $_tF_2 = N(\mu_2, \sigma^2)$. The null hypothesis is $H_0 : \mu_1 = \mu_2$, and the one-sided alternative $H_1 : \mu_1 > \mu_2$ is considered.

Being the common variance σ^2 unknown, it is estimated by the pooled variance estimator:

$$s_m^2 = \frac{s_{1,m_1}^2(m_1 - 1) + s_{2,m_2}^2(m_2 - 1)}{m_1 + m_2 - 2}$$

where the variance estimators of the two distributions are:

$$s_{i,m_i}^2 = \sum_{j=1}^{m_i}(X_{i,j} - \bar{X}_{i,m_i})^2/(m_i - 1), \qquad i = 1, 2$$

The test statistic is the standardized difference between the sample means:

$$T_m = \frac{\bar{X}_{1,m_1} - \bar{X}_{2,m_2}}{s_m\sqrt{\frac{1}{m_1} + \frac{1}{m_2}}} \tag{6.1}$$

Under the null hypothesis this T_m is distributed as a t with $m_1 + m_2 - 2$ dfs, i.e. $T_m \sim \tau_{m_1+m_2-2}$. The critical value of the test $t_{m,1-\alpha} = \tau_{m_1+m_2-2}^{-1}(1 - \alpha)$ is obtained and is to be used for defining the statistical test according to (5.1):

$$\psi_\alpha(T_m) = \begin{cases} 1 & \text{if} \quad T_m > \tau_{m_1+m_2-2}^{-1}(1 - \alpha) \\ 0 & \text{if} \quad T_m \leq \tau_{m_1+m_2-2}^{-1}(1 - \alpha) \end{cases} \tag{6.2}$$

The p-value, hence, is $1 - \tau_{m_1+m_2-2}(T_m)$.

6.1.1   Power and RP estimation

Under the alternative hypothesis, T_m has a noncentral t distribution with m_1+m_2-2 dfs, and with noncentrality parameter:

$$_t\lambda_m = \sqrt{m_1 m_2/(m_1 + m_2)}(\mu_1 - \mu_2)/\sigma$$

that is $T_m \sim \tau_{m_1+m_2-2,\,t\lambda_m}$. Being λ_m the generic noncentrality parameter, the power function, according to (5.3), is:

$$\pi(\alpha, \lambda_m) = 1 - \tau_{m_1+m_2-2,\lambda_m}\left(\tau_{m_1+m_2-2}^{-1}(1 - \alpha)\right)$$

When a sample of size n is given from $({}_tF_1, {}_tF_2)$, the γ lower bound for ${}_t\lambda_n$ (i.e. ℓ_n^γ) is obtained by the root of this equation, which is a particular case of (5.6):

$$\tau_{n_1+n_2-2,v}(T_n) = \gamma \tag{6.3}$$

According to (5.7) the RP estimator is thus:

$$\hat{RP}_\alpha^\gamma = 1 - \tau_{n_1+n_2-2,\ell_n^\gamma}(\tau_{n_1+n_2-2}^{-1}(1-\alpha))$$

which allows RP-testing as in (5.8).

6.1.2 Sample size estimation

The link function l is first needed to apply CSSE, and in this context it is $l(u_1, u_2) = \sqrt{u_1 u_2/(u_1 + u_2)}$. Then, $\ell_{m,n}^\gamma$ can be computed according to (5.10), and through (5.12) the γ-conservative sample size estimator is:

$$M_n^\gamma = \min\{m \quad : \quad 1 - \tau_{m_1+m_2-2,\ell_{m,n}^\gamma}(\tau_{m_1+m_2-2}^{-1}(1-\alpha)) > 1 - \beta\} \tag{6.4}$$

The launch criterion based on Clinical Relevance refers to the same effect size structure adopted when σ was known, i.e. $\delta_t = (\mu_1 - \mu_2)/\sigma$. It can, therefore, be expressed a launch threshold δ_{0L} to refer with in order to apply this launch criterion when the t-test is applied. In particular, $d_n = (\bar{X}_{1,n_1} - \bar{X}_{2,n_2})/s_n$ and $d_n^\gamma = \ell_n^\gamma/l(n)$ should be compared with δ_{0L}, for the PWS and the γ-CSSE strategies, respectively.

For this t-test, the OP in (5.13) can be approximated by the OP equation in case of known variance, that is, equation (3.17). In particular, d_n can be considered approximately normally distributed, with mean and variance equal to δ_t and $\frac{1}{n_1} + \frac{1}{n_2}$, respectively. Nevertheless, the OP in (5.13) can also be computed exactly on the basis of the distribution of $\ell_{m,n}^\gamma$, which can be derived starting from the fact that $\tau_{m_1+m_2-2,\ell_n^\gamma}^{-1}(\gamma) = T_n$ is distributed as a $\tau_{n_1+n_2-2,{}_t\lambda_n}$. However, the last part of the summand of the OP in (5.13) (i.e. $P(M_n^\gamma = m)$) cannot be written explicitly as in (3.14) of Section 3.5, and this is due to the dependence of the critical value of the test on m. $P(M_n^\gamma = m)$ should therefore be computed iteratively.

To apply COS, the OP has to be estimated. If the normal approximation of the OP is adopted, the estimated OP is obtained by plugging d_n in place of δ_t into (3.17). If the exact OP in (5.13) is considered, then ${}_t\lambda_m$ should be substituted by $\ell_{m,n} = \ell_n^{50\%}l(m)/l(n)$ in both parts of the summands of (5.13); in particular, $\ell_{m,n}$ should also be used to compute $P(M_n^\gamma = m)$. In both cases the estimated optimal conservativeness g_n^O is obtained in analogy with (3.21).

When it is postulated that the phase II effect size is different from that of phase III, a correction on the estimator of the latter effect size can be applied. Given the postulated correction k_c (which is defined in Section 4.3), the correction of the γ-conservative estimator of δ_t is $d_n^\gamma \times k_c = \ell_n^\gamma \times k_c/l(n)$. Consequently, the corrected estimator of $_t\lambda_m$ is $_c\ell^\gamma_{m,n} = \ell^\gamma_n \times k_c \times l(m)/l(n)$, and the sample size estimator is derived in analogy with the above formula on M^γ_n (i.e. (6.4)). The corrected COS follows from the estimation of the OP obtained in analogy with (4.5), where $\ell^{50\%}_n/l(n)$ plays the role of $d_{II,n}$, i.e. the estimator of the phase II effect size given by phase II data.

■ EXAMPLE 6.1

A phase II Randomized, Placebo-Controlled Clinical Trial on a new drug was conducted on two groups of size $n_1 = 23$ (drug) and $n_2 = 21$. The increase in a certain parameter of interest was, on average, $\bar{X}_{1,23} = 0.129$ and $\bar{X}_{2,21} = -0.004$, for the drug and the placebo groups, respectively. The estimated standard deviations were $s_{1,23} = 0.186$ and $s_{2,21} = 0.153$, giving a pooled estimate of $s_{(23,21)} = 0.171$. The observed effect size resulted, therefore, $d_{(23,21)} = (0.129 + 0.004)/0.171 = 0.7774$, where the test statistic $T_{(23,21)}$ was 2.576.

On this basis a new phase III trial was launched, and the PWS, 3QS and 1SES sample size estimates were computed, setting $\alpha = 2.5\%$ (one-tailed) and $1-\beta = 90\%$. At first, the estimates of the noncentrality parameter were derived, obtaining $\ell_{(23,21)} = 2.560$, $\ell^{75\%}_{(23,21)} = 1.860$ and $\ell^{84.1\%}_{(23,21)} = 1.523$. It is then easy to estimate $_t\lambda_m$, even conservatively, on the basis of $\ell^\bullet_{(23,21)}$ and of the link function $l()$. For a balanced design (i.e. $m_1 = m_2$) we have $l(m_1, m_2) = \sqrt{m_1/2}$. As a consequence, considering for example the PWS, we obtained $\ell_{(23,21);30} = l(30,30)\ell_{(23,21)}/l(23,21) = \sqrt{30/2} \times 2.560/\sqrt{23 \times 21/(23+21)} = 2.993$; as a further example $\ell_{(23,21);37} = 3.323$. Figure 6.1 reports the increasing estimates of the $SP(m)$, and it can be noted that the sample size estimates resulted $M_{(23,21)} = 37$, $M^{75\%}_{(23,21)} = 68$ and $M^{84.1\%}_{(23,21)} = 101$.

The sample size estimates for the unbalanced design with $m_1/m_2 = 2$ was also computed. Figure 6.2 reports the SP estimates for the smaller group (i.e. $SP(m_2)$), which gave $M_{(23,21)} = 28$, $M^{75\%}_{(23,21)} = 51$ and $M^{84.1\%}_{(23,21)} = 76$.

6.1.3 Final comments

The statistical test (6.2) is a superiority one, due to the definition of the test statistic T_m in (6.1). Nevertheless, (6.2) can be extended to clinic superiority and clinical non-inferiority by simply modifying T_m (see Section 1.8). Only the numerator in (6.1) should be changed, becoming $\bar{X}_{1,m_1} - \bar{X}_{2,m_2} - \delta_0$ when clinical superiority is under testing (i.e. $H_1 : \mu_1 > \mu_2 + \delta_0$) or $\bar{X}_{1,m_1} - \bar{X}_{2,m_2} + \delta_0$ for testing non-inferiority (i.e. $H_1 : \mu_1 > \mu_2 - \delta_0$). RP estimation and CSSE can be performed as explained in the two Subsections above.

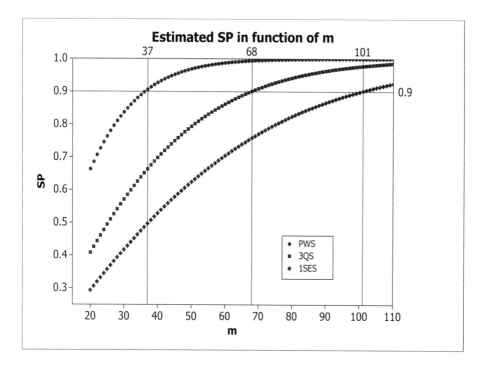

Figure 6.1 *PWS, 3QS and 1SES SP estimates for balanced designs, based on $n_1 = 23$ and $n_2 = 21$ phase II data of Example 6.1, in function of the phase III sample size m.*

6.2 Test for two means - unequal variances

The true distribution of the first population is assumed here to be $_tF_1 = N(\mu_1, \sigma_1^2)$, whereas the second one is $_tF_2 = N(\mu_2, \sigma_2^2)$. The hypotheses here considered are $H_0 : \mu_1 = \mu_2$, and $H_1 : \mu_1 > \mu_2$. Since the variances of the two populations were different, the pooled variance estimator is not adopted, and the test statistic is:

$$T_m = \frac{\bar{X}_{1,m_1} - \bar{X}_{2,m_2}}{\sqrt{\frac{s_{1,m_1}^2}{m_1} + \frac{s_{2,m_2}^2}{m_2}}}$$

T_m follows, approximately, a t-distribution with f dfs, where:

$$f = \frac{(\sigma_1^2/m_1 + \sigma_2^2/m_2)^2}{(\sigma_1^2/m_1)^2/(m_1 - 1) + (\sigma_2^2/m_2)^2/(m_2 - 1)}$$

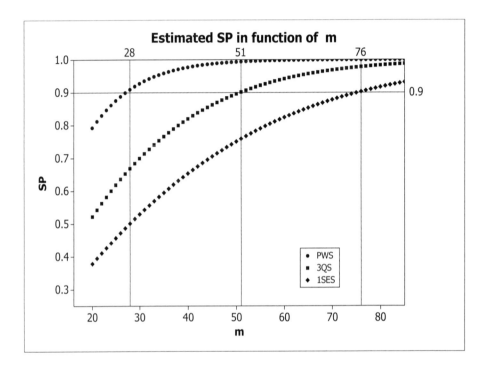

Figure 6.2 *PWS, 3QS and 1SES SP estimates for unbalanced designs (2:1), based on $n_1 = 23$ and $n_2 = 21$ phase II data of Example 6.1, in function of the phase III sample size m.*

This approximation of the distribution of T_m is due to the fact that the linear combination of variances under the square root of the denominator of T_m has an approximated χ^2 distribution. Moreover, note that the dfs are unknown, since f is a function of the unknown σ_i's. Then, f is, in practice, approximated by its estimate:

$$\hat{f} = \frac{(s_{1,m_1}^2/m_1 + s_{2,m_2}^2/m_2)^2}{(s_{1,m_1}^2/m_1)^2/(m_1 - 1) + (s_{2,m_2}^2/m_2)^2/(m_2 - 1)}$$

The critical value, therefore, becomes $t_{m,1-\alpha} = \tau_{\hat{f}}^{-1}(1 - \alpha)$. The statistical test, according to (5.1), is:

$$\psi_\alpha(T_m) = \begin{cases} 1 & \text{if} \quad T_m > \tau_{\hat{f}}^{-1}(1 - \alpha) \\ 0 & \text{if} \quad T_m \leq \tau_{\hat{f}}^{-1}(1 - \alpha) \end{cases} \tag{6.5}$$

and the p-value results $1 - \tau_{\hat{f}}(T_m)$. This testing procedure is also known as the Welch test (see Welch, 1947, 1949). Only it should be noted that the actual probability of the type I error does not coincide with α, since T_m has an approximated t distribution. In other words, this is not an exact test.

6.2.1 Power and RP estimation

Here, the noncentrality parameter is $_t\lambda_m = (\mu_1 - \mu_2)/\sqrt{\sigma_1^2/m_1 + \sigma_2^2/m_2}$ (see, for example, Scheffé, 1970). For this unequal variances t-test the power definition, the noncentral parameter estimation, the RP estimation and the RP-testing are analogous to that of the equal variances t-test (Section 6.1.1).

Since T_m is approximately distributed as a Student's t, the power function is an approximation and it does not report the exact power.

EXAMPLE 6.2

In a phase III randomized, controlled clinical trial a new treatment was compared with a standard control, and the type I error probability was set at 1%, one-tailed. Two groups of size $n_1 = 60$ and $n_2 = 62$ were drawn up. The variables of primary interest, i.e. the pre-post differences of a certain clinical parameter, showed Gaussian shapes and different standard deviations: $s_{1,60} = 3.467$ and $s_{2,62} = 1.029$. Moreover, the new treatment performed better than the control, the trial providing $\bar{X}_{1,60} = 5.178$ versus $\bar{X}_{2,62} = 3.283$.

The test statistic resulted, therefore, $T_{(60,62)} = 4.064$, with an estimated amount of 69 dfs (actually, $\hat{f} = 69.00298$). The p-value, hence, was lower than 10^{-4} (i.e. $1 - \tau_{69}(4.064) = 0.00006$; compare with Table A.3). The pointwise RP resulted 94.97%, where the conservative estimates provided $\hat{RP}_{1\%}^{90\%} = 62.35\%$ and $\hat{RP}_{1\%}^{95\%} = 47.54\%$. This statistical significance was to be considered G-stable, 90%-stable and almost 95%-stable.

6.2.2 Sample size estimation

In order to derive $\ell_{m,n}^\gamma$ from ℓ_n^γ, due to the difference of the variances, a constraint about the rate between the sample size of the two groups should be introduced. Let us assume that $c = n_2/n_1 = m_2/m_1$. Then, ℓ_n^γ estimates $_t\lambda_n = \sqrt{n_1}(\mu_1 - \mu_2)/\sqrt{\sigma_1^2 + \sigma_2^2/c}$ which depends on n_1 only. The link function is therefore $l(u_1, u_2) = \sqrt{u_1}$, which provides $\ell_{m,n}^\gamma = \ell_n^\gamma \sqrt{m_1}/\sqrt{n_1}$. Then, the sample size estimator formula (6.4) remains valid.

According to previous definitions of the standardized effect size, here δ_t seems to be represented by $(\mu_1 - \mu_2)/\sqrt{(\sigma_1^2 + \sigma_2^2/c)/2}$. It is worth noting that the balancing of sampling (i.e. the value of c) affects this standardized value. This result is ambiguous since the effect size should depend only on the distributions F_1 and F_2, not on the design. For this reason, in this context avoidance of the launching criterion based on the effect size and the adoption of one of the other two criteria is suggested. Only when the allocation of treatments is balanced, i.e. $c = 1$, this effect size does not depend on c and it can therefore be considered for launching purposes. In this case see Section 6.1.2.

As far as OP computations are concerned, they can be performed only approximately, either referring to the normal approximation, or to the t one (remember that T_m has an approximated t distribution). In the former case, the role of d_n is played by $(\bar{X}_{1,n_1} - \bar{X}_{2,n_2})/\sqrt{(s_{1,n_1}^2 + s_{2,n_2}^2/c)/2}$ and the distribution of this quantity is approximated by a Gaussian with mean and variance equal, respectively, to $(\mu_1 - \mu_2)/\sqrt{(\sigma_1^2 + \sigma_2^2/c)/2}$ and $2/n_1$. If the approximation to the t is adopted, then the computation of $P(M_n^\gamma = m)$ can not be performed directly (as for the t-test with equal variances), but it can either be done iteratively or through simulation.

To apply COS, the (normally) approximated OP can be estimated by plugging the estimator $(\bar{X}_{1,n_1} - \bar{X}_{2,n_2})/\sqrt{(s_{1,n_1}^2 + s_{2,n_2}^2/c)/2}$ into (3.17) in place of δ_t, and the optimal amount of conservativeness g_n^O can be derived from (3.21).

6.2.3 Final comments

Also this unequal variances t-test can be extended for evaluating clinical superiority and clinical non-inferiority, in analogy with the previous t-test: the numerator of the test statistic can be modified - see Section 6.1.3.

In order to obtain a test statistic with exact t distribution even when the variances of the two groups are unequal, an experimental design different from the two parallel arms here considered should be adopted. For example, a matched-pair parallel design or a 2×2 crossover design may be adopted (see Shao and Chow, 2002). In these situations, the SP can be estimated using the techniques shown in Section 6.1.

6.3 On Student's t RP estimates

It is worth noting that with small p-values RP estimates given by t distributions are a bit higher than the corresponding ones when the distribution of the test statistic is Gaussian. For example, the corresponding RP estimates given by the Gaussian approximation of the distribution of $T_{(60,62)}$, in relation to the observed value of 4.064 of Example 6.2 would have been 93.42%, 58.96% and 44.56%, with $\gamma = 50\%, 90\%, 95\%$, respectively, where those given by the t distribution were 94.97%, 62.35%, 47.54%. As the dfs increase the difference between RP estimates decreases.

In order to show a comparison of the behavior of RP estimates in the following Figure 6.3 we reported the RP curves with $\gamma = 50\%, 90\%, 95\%$ for the t distribution with

30 dfs together with the corresponding ones for the Gaussian distribution, already shown in Figure 2.5 ($\alpha = 2.5\%$, one-tailed).

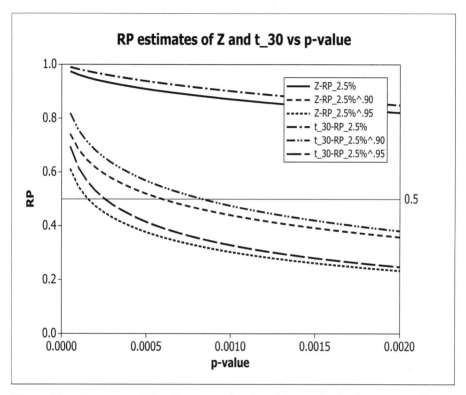

Figure 6.3   *Conservative RP estimates as a function of the p-value for the t-test, in relation with those of the Z-test. The one-tailed setting is considered, with $\alpha = 2.5\%$.*

CHAPTER 7

SP ESTIMATION FOR GAUSSIAN DISTRIBUTED TEST STATISTICS

This Chapter considers SP estimation for tests whose distribution function of the generic test statistic, i.e. G_{m,λ_m}, is a Gaussian with mean λ_m and unitary variance: $G_{m,\lambda_m} = \Phi_{\lambda_m,1}$.

Two tests are studied, whose actual test statistic is approximately Gaussian distributed. The first test concerns the comparison between two proportions from different populations, which is sometimes called the "large sample test for proportions". Then, a problem in survival analysis is discussed, considering the so-called "log-rank test", which compares two survival curves.

7.1 Test for two proportions

It is interesting to compare the proportions p_1 and p_2 of a certain feature in two different populations. The outcomes are of the yes/no type and if they are coded as $1/0$, then the elements of the two samples X_{ij} have a Bernoullian distribution with parameters p_i, $i = 1, 2$. In other words, X_{ij} have distributions $_tF_i = Ber(p_i)$, where $P(X_{ij} = 1) = p_i$. The null hypothesis considered here is that of no difference

Success Probability Estimation with Applications to Clinical Trials, First Edition.
By Daniele De Martini Copyright © 2013 John Wiley & Sons, Inc.

between proportions: $H_0 : p_1 = p_2$, and the test for the one-sided alternative $H_1 :$ $p_1 > p_2$ is developed.

The sample frequencies $\hat{p}_{i,m_i} = \#\{X_{ij} = 1\}/m_i$ form the basis when building the test statistic, which is the standardized difference between them. Since $Var(\hat{p}_{i,m_i}) = p_i(1 - p_i)/m_i$, T_m results:

$$T_m = \frac{\hat{p}_{1,m_1} - \hat{p}_{2,m_2}}{\sqrt{\hat{p}_{1,m_1}(1 - \hat{p}_{1,m_1})/m_1 + \hat{p}_{2,m_2}(1 - \hat{p}_{2,m_2})/m_2}}$$

Noting that the sample frequencies can be viewed as sample means, i.e. $\hat{p}_{i,m_i} = \sum_{j=1}^{m_i} X_{ij}/m_i$, $i = 1, 2$, through the application of the Central Limit Theorem (see, for example, Lehmann and Romano, 2005) it is easy to obtain that the distribution of T_m can be approximated by a normal distribution.

Under the null hypothesis, T_m is approximately distributed as a standard normal $N(0, 1)$, so that the critical value of the test (5.1) is $t_{m,1-\alpha} = \Phi^{-1}(1 - \alpha) = z_{1-\alpha}$ and the test results:

$$\psi_\alpha(T_m) = \begin{cases} 1 & \text{if} \quad T_m > z_{1-\alpha} \\ 0 & \text{if} \quad T_m \le z_{1-\alpha} \end{cases} \tag{7.1}$$

The p-value is $1 - \Phi(T_m)$. The actual probability of the type I error of the test is just close to α, not equal to it, since the distribution of T_m is not exactly Gaussian. Consequently, this is not an exact test.

The approximation of T_m to the Gaussian is good if m is sufficiently large *and* the p_i's are not too close to the limits of their range, i.e. 0 and 1. A high sample size alone is not sufficient. As a consequence, even when the sample size is considered high enough (e.g. 20) the actual type I error can be quite a bit higher than α. For example, Eberhardt and Fligner (1977, p. 155) reported a situation where the level was more than 8% with $\alpha = 5\%$ and $m_1 = m_2 = 20$.

In fact, the approximation of T_m to the Gaussian is based on the approximation of the binomial distribution to the latter. A simple rule of thumb is that $m_i p_i$ and $m_i(1 - p_i)$ should be greater than 5. Nevertheless, this threshold depends on the goodness of the approximation desired, and for this reason on some other occasions the suggested threshold was 10. Some other approximation rules can be found in the literature (e.g. see Box et al., 2005).

7.1.1   Power and RP estimation

Under the alternative, T_m is approximately distributed as a Gaussian with unitary variance and mean $_t\lambda_m$ (i.e. $\simeq N(_t\lambda_m, 1)$), where:

$$_t\lambda_m = (p_1 - p_2)/\sqrt{p_1(1 - p_1)/m_1 + p_2(1 - p_2)/m_2}$$

Considering the generic distributions $F_1 = Ber(p')$ and $F_2 = Ber(p'')$, the generic noncentrality parameter is $\lambda_m = (p' - p'')/\sqrt{p'(1 - p')/m_1 + p''(1 - p'')/m_2}$. Therefore, the approximated power function is:

$$\pi(\alpha, \lambda_m) = \Phi(\lambda_m - z_{1-\alpha})$$

giving:

$$SP = \Phi(_t\lambda_m - z_{1-\alpha})$$

When a sample of size n is given, the lower bounds for $_t\lambda_n$ can be obtained according to (5.6), resulting $\ell_n^\gamma = T_n - z_\gamma$. The estimator of SP at the size $m = n$ assumes the meaning of RP which, therefore, results:

$$\hat{RP}_\alpha^\gamma = \Phi(T_n - z_\gamma - z_{1-\alpha})$$

In this case, although the power is approximated, the RP-test (5.8) holds exactly, in the sense that it is equivalent to (7.1). As a consequence, neither test is exact.

7.1.2 Sample size estimation

In analogy with the situation of Section 6.2, where the variances were unequal, in order to perform CSSE based on the derivation of $\ell_{m,n}^\gamma$ from ℓ_n^γ, the first assumption is that there is a fixed rate between the sample sizes of the two groups: $c = n_2/n_1$. (Note that c can eventually be chosen in order to improve the power of the test, as shown in Brittain and Schlesselman, 1982). Then, the lower bound for the noncentrality parameter given by pilot data (i.e. ℓ_n^γ), regarding sample sizes, depends only on n_1, not on n_2. Consequently the analogous estimator of the noncentrality parameter at size m can be obtained through (5.10) with the link function l applied only to n_1 and m_1, obviously when the balancing c is maintained (i.e. $c = m_2/m_1$). In practice, since $l(u) = \sqrt{u_1}$ we have $\ell_{m,n}^\gamma = \ell_n^\gamma \sqrt{m_1}/\sqrt{n_1}$. The application of (5.12) to estimate M_I conservatively gives, for the first group:

$$M_{n,1}^\gamma = \left\lfloor \frac{(z_{1-\alpha} + z_{1-\beta})^2}{\left(\frac{\hat{p}_{1,n_1} - \hat{p}_{2,n_2}}{\sqrt{\hat{p}_{1,n_1}(1 - \hat{p}_{1,n_1}) + \hat{p}_{2,n_2}(1 - \hat{p}_{2,n_2})/c}} - z_\gamma/\sqrt{n_1} \right)^2} \right\rfloor + 1$$

As far as the launch criterion based on the clinical relevance is concerned, the analogous of the standardized effect size $\delta_t = (\mu_1 - \mu_2)/\sigma$ should firstly be defined in this context. The difference between the proportions is to be taken into account, and to be related to the population standard deviations (i.e. $\sqrt{p_i(1 - p_i)}$, $i = 1, 2$). So, $(p_1 - p_2)/\sqrt{(p_1(1 - p_1) + p_2(1 - p_2)/c)/2}$ should be considered as the true effect size. Nevertheless, in analogy with Section 6.2.2 where two means with unknown unequal variances were compared, this effect size is ambiguous since it contains the rate c of balancing. Then, the adoption of another launching criterion is suggested.

Table 7.1   Amplitude of the generic effect sizes for binomial comparisons under balanced sampling. p_m stands for $\min\{p'', 1 - p'\}$.

| | Amplitude of effect size $\delta(p)$ | | | | | | | | | |
| | $p' - p''$ | | | | | | | | | |
	0.05	0.1	0.15	0.2	0.25	0.3	0.35	0.4	0.45	0.5
p_m										
0.05	0.19	0.34	0.47	0.58	0.70	0.81	0.92	1.04	1.17	1.30
0.1	0.15	0.28	0.40	0.52	0.63	0.74	0.85	0.97	1.10	1.23
0.15	0.13	0.25	0.37	0.47	0.58	0.69	0.81	0.92	1.05	1.19
0.2	0.12	0.23	0.34	0.45	0.55	0.66	0.78	0.89	1.02	1.16
0.25	0.11	0.22	0.32	0.43	0.53	0.64	0.76	0.88	1.01	1.15
0.3	0.11	0.21	0.31	0.42	0.52	0.63	0.75	0.87	-	-
0.35	0.10	0.21	0.31	0.41	0.52	0.63	-	-	-	-
0.4	0.10	0.20	0.30	0.41	-	-	-	-	-	-
0.45	0.10	0.20	-	-	-	-	-	-	-	-

When the design is balanced (i.e. $c = 1$) the quantity playing the role of the true effect size δ_t is independent of c, since it becomes

$$\delta(p_t) = (p_1 - p_2)/\sqrt{(p_1(1 - p_1) + p_2(1 - p_2))/2}$$

where $p_t = (p_1, p_2)$. The launch threshold based on clinical relevance might in this case be adopted, and we suggest that reference be made to the order of magnitude for δ_{0L} that has already been assimilated in Chapter 3. Consequently, the values of the generic $\delta(p)$ are provided in Table 7.1 for some values of $p = (p', p'')$. For example, if one intends the minimum difference between proportions in order to launch to be $p' - p'' = 0.1$ and assumes a p'' of 0.7, then $\min\{p'', 1 - p'\} = 0.2$ and the effect size (fourth line, second column) is $\delta(p) = 0.23$.

The OP defined in (3.12) can be computed as a function of the conservative parameter γ by referring to (3.17), since the normal approximation can be exploited. In particular, $(p_1 - p_2)/\sqrt{(p_1(1 - p_1) + p_2(1 - p_2)/c)/2}$ plays the role of the effect size δ_t.

In order to apply the COS, when two pilot samples give $\hat{p}_n = (\hat{p}_{1,n_1}, \hat{p}_{2,n_2})$, it is worth noting that:

$$\delta(\hat{p}_n) = (\hat{p}_{1,n_1} - \hat{p}_{2,n_2})/\sqrt{(\hat{p}_{1,n_1}(1 - \hat{p}_{1,n_1}) + \hat{p}_{2,n_2}(1 - \hat{p}_{2,n_2})/c)/2}$$

plays here the role of the estimator of the effect size d_n of Chapter 3. Then, $\delta(\hat{p}_n)$ can be plugged into (3.17) in place of δ_t to obtain an estimator of the OP. Finally, the optimal g_n^O can be computed as in (3.21).

Assuming that the phase II effect size is different from that of the phase III, under the balanced sampling (i.e. $c = 1$) the correction on the effect size estimator $\delta(\hat{p}_n)$ can be applied. Given, therefore, the postulated correction to be applied (i.e. k_c), the corrected γ-conservative estimator of $_t\lambda_m$ is $\ell_{m,n}^\gamma \times k_c = (\delta(\hat{p}_n)/\sqrt{2} - z_\gamma/\sqrt{n_1})k_c\sqrt{m_1}$. Then, the corrected sample size estimator for each group is

$$_cM_n^\gamma = \lfloor 2(z_{1-\alpha} + z_{1-\beta})^2/((\delta(\hat{p}_n) - z_\gamma/\sqrt{n_1/2})k_c)^2 \rfloor + 1$$

The correction of the effect size can also be applied to COS by exploiting (4.5), where $\delta(\hat{p}_n) = T_n\sqrt{2/n_1}$ is used in place of $d_{II,n}$.

7.1.3 Final comments

Some exact statistical tests for comparing two proportions have been proposed over the years, starting from Fisher (1922). Their computation, however, is often complicated. Agresti (1992) provides a useful survey of these tests, and Berger (1996) presents a solution based on confidence interval p-value which is often more powerful than the test based on asymptotic normality (i.e. (7.1)).

As far as their (exact) power function is concerned, it should be noted that they do not depend only on the difference between the two proportions, but also on the positions of the latter in the range $(0, 1)$. Consequently, the power functions of these exact tests do not fall under the general formula (5.3) (whereas the approximated test (7.1) does) and their SPs cannot, therefore, be estimated by referring to the techniques disclosed in this Chapter. Nevertheless, SP estimation for exact tests can be performed following the general nonparametric method that will be introduced in Chapter 9.

7.2 Test for survival: the log-rank test

When the survival rates over time of the two populations are to be compared, the log-rank test can be applied. The data of the two samples (i.e. the X_{ij}) are, in this context, bivariate. Not only the duration of the observation (i.e. the survival time) of the patients should be considered, but also if the end of the observation has been caused by death or by so-called censoring. In practice the duration of the observation is called *censored* when the end-point of interest (i.e. dead) has not been observed. This can be due either to the fact that the patient has been lost to follow-up (for example because he moved to another country) or because the patient is still alive at the end of the trial. So, the first component of X_{ij} (i.e. $X_{ij,1}$) represents the duration of the observation of the patient, where $X_{ij,2}$ is equal to 0 in case of dead and to 1 when the observation is censored. To be precise, X_{ij} belongs to the space $R^+ \times \{0, 1\}$.

According to Section 7.1, the data X_{ij}'s, $j = 1, \ldots, m_i$, follow the distributions $_tF_i$, $i = 1, 2$. The null hypothesis is that the distributions of the survival times are equal: $H_0 : {}_tF_1 = {}_tF_2$. Often, the alternative considered is two-sided, i.e. $H_1 : {}_tF_1 \neq {}_tF_2$; nevertheless, it is also possible to build the test for the one-sided alternative.

In order to build the test statistic T_m some notations should be introduced. Consider just the times of the deaths, that are $X_{ij,1}$ such that the corresponding $X_{ij,2} = 0$, and sort these times denoting them by $t_1 < t_2 < \cdots < t_r$. Usually $r < m_1 + m_2$, and there is equality only when all the times are different and there are no censored observations.

For each one of the uncensored times, the number of potential deaths, i.e. the number of patients still alive immediately before the observational time, is counted together with the number of actual deaths at that time, for each group. In formulas, for the first group the above quantities result: $n_{1k} = \#\{X_{1j} \text{ such that } X_{1j,1} \geq t_k\}$, and $d_{1k} = \#\{X_{1j} \text{ such that } X_{1j,1} = t_k \text{ and } X_{1j,2} = 0\}$, for $k = 1, \ldots, r$. n_{2k} and d_{2k} are computed analogously using the control sample. The total number of patients and of observed deaths at time k are, therefore, $n_k = n_{1k} + n_{2k}$ and $d_k = d_{1k} + d_{2k}$, respectively.

Then, the expected number of deaths at time k for the first group (i.e. e_{1k}) is given by the number of patients alive at time k in the first group times the proportion of deaths at time k over all groups, that is $e_{1k} = n_{1k}d_k/n_k$. Analogously e_{2k} is built. Consequently, the differences between the expected and the observed number of deaths for all the times (i.e. e_{ik} and d_{ik} for $k = 1, \ldots, r$) represent the basis to build the test statistic. It is intuitive that it is sufficient to focus on one group only, and it is usual to do this on the first one. So, the sum of the differences is considered: $U = \sum_{k=1}^{r}(d_{1k} - e_{1k})$.

Under the null hypothesis the rate of deaths of each group should be equal at each time; consequently, the differences $d_{ik} - e_{ik}$ have mean equal to 0, and so also U has mean 0. Moreover, U has on approximated normal distribution, when r (viz. the times of deaths) is sufficiently large. Finally, the variance of U is $V = \sum_{k=1}^{r} n_{1k}n_{2k}d_k(n_k - d_k)/n_k^2(n_k - 1)$.

Hence, the test statistic:

$$T_m = U/\sqrt{V}$$

under the null hypothesis follows, approximately, a standard normal distribution. Once α has been set, due to the two-sided alternative in H_1, the critical values are $\Phi^{-1}(\alpha/2) = z_{\alpha/2}$ and $\Phi^{-1}(1 - \alpha/2) = z_{1-\alpha/2}$, so that the test is:

$$\psi_\alpha(T_m) = \begin{cases} 1 & \text{if} \quad T_m < z_{\alpha/2} \text{ or } T_m > z_{1-\alpha/2} \\ 0 & \text{if} \quad z_{\alpha/2} \leq T_m \leq z_{1-\alpha/2} \end{cases} \tag{7.2}$$

Highly negative values of T_m (i.e. lower than $z_{\alpha/2}$) report that the number of deaths from $_tF_1$ is lower than expected under the null and so represent experimental proof that the new drug is effective with respect to the control one. For this two-tailed test the p-value is $2(1 - \Phi(|T_m|))$, in analogy with (1.16).

7.2.1   Power and RP estimation

Under the alternative T_m has approximately a normal distribution with unitary variance and mean (i.e. the noncentrality parameter) $_t\lambda_m$. To explain the structure of this $_t\lambda_m$ some other concepts related to survival modeling, such as the survivor function and the hazard function, should be introduced (for further readings in survival analysis one can see Collett, 2003). Moreover, the meaning of $_t\lambda_m$ depends on the model assumptions (see Zhang and Quan, 2009).

Nevertheless, due to the approximated normality of the test statistic, given a sample of size n it is possible to compute conservative estimates of $_t\lambda_n$ and to apply RP estimation and stability evaluations for the two-tailed setting in analogy with Section 2.9. In particular, recall that $\hat{RP}_{2;\alpha}^{\gamma} = \Phi(|T_m| - z_\gamma - z_{1-\alpha/2})$. Then, the RP-test in (5.8), where $\hat{RP}_{2;\alpha}^{50\%} = \hat{RP}_{2;\alpha}$ is used, is equivalent to the latter, i.e. (7.2).

▐ EXAMPLE 7.1

In order to evaluate a new drug for patients affected by a certain illness, a comparative phase III trial with a standard control drug has been conducted over two groups of patients of sizes $n_1 = 103$ and $n_2 = 101$, respectively. A survival analysis at 5 years has been performed, Kaplan-Meier survival curves are reported in Figure 7.1, and the log-rank test has been applied. The type I error was set at 5% and the test statistic provided by the experimental data was $T_{(103,101)} = -2.728$, so that the two-tailed p-value resulted 0.00636 (see Table A.1). The two-tailed pointwise RP (i.e. $\hat{RP}_{2;5\%}$) resulted 77.90%, where the conservative estimates provided $\hat{RP}_{2;5\%}^{90\%} = 30.40\%$ and $\hat{RP}_{2;5\%}^{95\%} = 19.05\%$ (use Tables B.4-B.6). So, although the study showed a significant result (actually, a (**) moderate one) in favor of the new drug, the experimental proof was not stable enough.

7.2.2   Sample size estimation

The sample size M_I can be estimated on the basis of an n sized sample, once model assumptions that generate $_t\lambda_m$ have been set. Although different models provide different structures of $_t\lambda_m$, equal values of the latter induced by different models provide equal SP and M_I. Analogously, whatever the model is, given the pilot sample, the estimate of $_t\lambda_n$ is uniquely determined. Nevertheless, in order to estimate

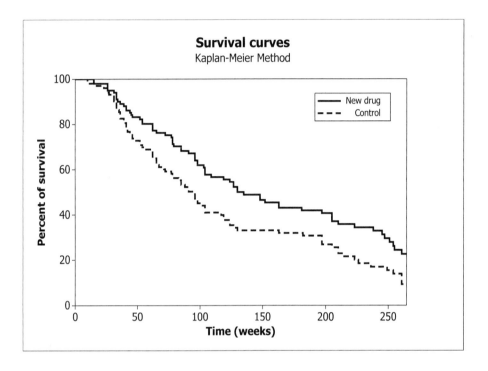

Figure 7.1   *Kaplan-Meier 5 years survival curves of the two groups of $n_1 = 103$ and $n_2 = 101$ patients of Example 7.1.*

M_I through (5.12), the link function l introduced in Section 5.3 is needed to compute $\ell^\gamma_{m,n}$. It should be noted that often (i.e. with some different models) l turns out to be $l(u) = \sqrt{u_1 + u_2}$ (Zhang and Quan, 2009).

Then, the γ-conservative estimator of M_I of the first group, provided that $\ell^\gamma_n = T_n - z_\gamma > 0$, is:

$$M^\gamma_{n,1} = \left\lfloor \frac{(z_{1-\alpha} + z_{1-\beta})^2 (n_1 + n_2)}{(T_n - z_\gamma)^2 (1 + c)} \right\rfloor + 1$$

where $c = m_2/m_1$.

Due to the difficulty in defining and understanding the meaning of the noncentrality parameter that is linked to the effect size, the launching criteria of statistical significance of phase II data or that based on the maximum sample size for the phase III should be adopted in this context.

7.2.3 Final comments

Another statistical test for comparing survival data was proposed by Breslow (1970), and is also known as Wilcoxon test for survival (see Collett, 2003, for a comparison among the log-rank and the Wilcoxon tests for survival). Further, Jennrich (1984) introduced some exact tests for comparing survival curves in the presence of right censoring. The estimation of the RP and the sample size for these tests may be done using ad-hoc procedures, or also by applying the general technique for SP estimation that will be introduced in Chapter 9.

CHAPTER 8

SP ESTIMATION FOR CHI-SQUARE STATISTICAL TESTS

In this Chapter, two tests are considered for SP estimation, both based on contingency tables. Here, G_{m,λ_m} is a χ^2 distribution with C degrees of freedom and noncentrality parameter λ_m, that is $G_{m,\lambda_m} = \chi^2_{C-1,\lambda_m}$.

First, the test for comparing the outcomes of a categorical variable in two populations is studied. Then, the problem of comparing two proportions over a certain number of strata is considered, and the so-called Mantel-Haenszel test is adopted.

8.1 Test for two multinomial distributions: $2 \times C$ comparative trial

Let's now focus on categorical data with C different categories. Consider the m_1 sized sample from the first population (i.e. X_{1j}, $j = 1, \ldots, m_1$) and the m_2 sized one from the second population (i.e. X_{2j}, $j = 1, \ldots, m_2$) falling into C different categories. For each group there is a specific probability to fall into the generic category h: $P(X_{ij} = h) = \pi_{i,h}$ for each j, with $h = 1, \ldots, C$, $i = 1, 2$. These probabilities are collected in two vectors $\pi_i = (\pi_{i,1}, \ldots, \pi_{i,C})$, $i = 1, 2$, whose sums are equal to 1 in each group, i.e. $\sum_{h=1}^{C} \pi_{1,h} = \sum_{h=1}^{C} \pi_{2,h} = 1$. In other words,

Success Probability Estimation with Applications to Clinical Trials, First Edition.
By Daniele De Martini Copyright © 2013 John Wiley & Sons, Inc.

the random variables X_{ij} have multinomial distribution $_tF_i = \pi_i$, $j = 1, \ldots, m_i$, $i = 1, 2$.

The null hypothesis is that there is no difference between $_tF_1$ and $_tF_2$, that is, between the two vectors of probabilities: $H_0 : \pi_1 = \pi_2$, whereas the alternative is that there are some differences: $H_1 : \pi_1 \neq \pi_2$.

In order to build the test statistic, let us now consider the sample counts of the i-th group in the h-th category: $m_{i,h} = (\#X_{ij} = h)$. Then, let $p_{i,h} = m_{i,h}/m_i$ be the sample frequencies of the i-th group (also known as conditional proportions), that have total sum equal to 1: $\sum_{h=1}^{C} p_{i,h} = 1$, $i = 1, 2$. Under H_0 the two vectors π_i's are equal, and so it makes sense to provide a single estimator of the proportion for the h-th category, that is $p_{\bullet,h} = (m_{1,h} + m_{2,h})/(m_1 + m_2)$.

The test statistic is, hence, based on the $2 \times C$ differences between the observed frequencies (i.e. $p_{i,h}$) and the frequencies expected under the null (i.e. $p_{\bullet,h}$). In particular, the weighted sum of the standardized squared differences is computed, and so:

$$T_m = \sum_{i=1}^{2} \sum_{h=1}^{C} \frac{(p_{i,h} - p_{\bullet,h})^2}{p_{\bullet h}} \times m_i$$

This test statistic can be formulated also on the basis of counts $m_{i,h}$, that is:

$$T_m = \sum_{i=1}^{2} \sum_{h=1}^{C} \frac{\left(m_{i,h} - \frac{(m_{1,h}+m_{2,h})m_i}{m_1+m_2}\right)^2}{\frac{(m_{1,h}+m_{2,h})m_i}{m_1+m_2}}$$

Under H_0, T_m is asymptotically (i.e. as m increases) distributed as a χ^2 with $C - 1$ dfs, whose cumulative distribution is denoted by χ^2_{C-1}. The critical value is, therefore, $t_{m,1-\alpha} = {\chi^2_{C-1}}^{-1}(1 - \alpha)$, so that the statistical test (5.1) becomes:

$$\psi_\alpha(T_m) = \begin{cases} 1 & \text{if} \quad T_m > {\chi^2_{C-1}}^{-1}(1 - \alpha) \\ 0 & \text{if} \quad T_m \leq {\chi^2_{C-1}}^{-1}(1 - \alpha) \end{cases} \qquad (8.1)$$

The p-value of this test is $1 - \chi^2_{C-1}(T_m)$, according to (5.2).

8.1.1   Power and RP estimation

Under the alternative hypothesis, T_m has, approximately, a noncentral χ^2 distribution with $C - 1$ dfs and with noncentrality parameter:

$$_t\lambda_m = m_1 m_2/(m_1 + m_2) \sum_{h=1}^{C} (\pi_{1,h} - \pi_{2,h})^2/\pi_{2,h}$$

Table 8.1 Classification of the phase III outcomes of the variable of primary interest in the Treatment and in the Control group of Example 8.1.

	1	2	3	4	
Treatment	5	16	58	59	138
	3.62%	11.59%	42.03%	42.75%	
Control	19	22	57	35	133
	14.29%	16.54%	42.86%	26.32%	

(see Lachin, 1977). Formally, we have $T_m \simeq \chi^2_{C-1,\,t\lambda_m}$. According to (5.3), and being λ_m the generic noncentrality parameter, the approximated power function is

$$\pi(\alpha, \lambda_m) = 1 - \chi^2_{C-1,\lambda_m}\left(\chi^{2\,-1}_{C-1}(1-\alpha)\right)$$

Given a sample of size n, the γ lower bound for $_t\lambda_n$ (i.e. ℓ_n^γ) can be computed: it is provided by the root v of the following equation, according to (5.6):

$$\chi^2_{C-1,v}(T_n) = \gamma \tag{8.2}$$

The γ-conservative RP estimator can now be defined, resulting:

$$\hat{RP}_\alpha^\gamma = 1 - \chi^2_{C-1,\ell_n^\gamma}\left(\chi^{2\,-1}_{C-1}(1-\alpha)\right)$$

When the pointwise RP estimator $\hat{RP}_\alpha = \hat{RP}_\alpha^{50\%}$ is adopted, the RP-test (as in (5.8)) provides equal results to the above test (8.1).

◼ EXAMPLE 8.1

In a phase III trial a new treatment was tested to verify if the distribution of a four-classes categorical variable (viz. $C = 4$) had been modified with respect to that provided by a classical control drug. The four levels indicate the increasing degree of improvement of patient conditions. α was set at 2.5%, and a total of 271 patients were recruited, 138 of which underwent the new treatment (133 under control). The observed outcomes are reported in Table 8.1 and it is easy to note that the distribution of the new treatment is denser on higher columns.

The χ^2 test statistic resulted 15.163, giving a p-value of 0.00168, since it referred to a distribution with $(4 - 1) = 3$ dfs (see also Table A.4). Although the result is (**) significant, and the pointwise RP estimate resulted quite high (i.e. $\hat{RP}_{2.5\%} = 80.84\%$), it is not stable. Indeed, the 90%-conservative estimate of the RP resulted $\hat{RP}_{2.5\%}^{90\%} = 34.60\%$ ($\hat{RP}_{2.5\%}^{95\%} = 22.58\%$), that is below the *threshold of significance for the RP of $1/2$. The observed statistically significant result is therefore not 90%-stable.*

8.1.2 Sample size estimation

Here, the link function l is the square of that of the t-test with equal variances: $l(u) = u_1 u_2/(u_1 + u_2)$. According to (5.10) the lower bound for $_t\lambda_m$ is therefore $\ell_{m,n}^\gamma = \ell_n^\gamma m_1 m_2 (n_1 + n_2)/n_1 n_2 (m_1 + m_2)$. Through (5.12) it is found that:

$$M_n^\gamma = \min\{m \quad : \quad 1 - \chi^2_{C-1,\ell_{m,n}^\gamma}(\chi^2_{C-1}{}^{-1}(1 - \alpha)) > 1 - \beta\} \tag{8.3}$$

Regarding the launch criterion based on clinical relevance, the effect size is, in this context, difficult to interpret from a clinical perspective. Several authors (e.g. Cohen, 1988) indicate $\sqrt{T_m/m}$ as an effect size measure, i.e. an estimate of the effect size, when two multinomial distributions are compared. Further discussion on effect size for contingency tables can be found in Rosenthal (1994) and in McCartney and Rosenthal (2000). Some classifications of this effect size can also be found in the literature, but their clinical meaning is of concern. The adoption of one of the other two launching criteria of Section 3.3 is therefore suggested.

The OP is computed as in (5.13). Regarding the computation of $P(M_n^\gamma = m)$, the distribution of M_n^γ can be derived exactly. Starting from (8.2) and inverting both terms of the equivalence it is found that $\chi^2_{C-1,\ell_n^\gamma}{}^{-1}(\gamma) = T_n$ is distributed as a noncentral χ^2 with $C - 1$ dfs and noncentrality parameter $_t\lambda_n$. Then, due to the monotonicity of $g(v) = \chi^2_{C-1,v}{}^{-1}(\gamma)$, also the distribution of ℓ_n^γ is well defined, and it can be derived at least numerically. Consequently, the distribution of $\chi^2_{C-1,\ell_{m,n}^\gamma}(\chi^2_{C-1}{}^{-1}(1 - \alpha))$ can be computed and, finally, also that of M_n^γ.

In order to apply COS the OP has to be estimated, and its estimate can be computed by plugging ℓ_n in place of $_t\lambda_n$ in (5.13). In practice, the computational procedure of the OP explained above should be applied considering ℓ_n as if it were the true noncentrality parameter. Then, g_n^O is obtained in analogy with (3.21).

■ **EXAMPLE 8.2**

At the end of a phase II trial the categorical outcomes of the primary variable given by two groups (treatment and control) of $n_1 = n_2 = 61$ patients are resumed in the contingency Table 8.2.

It is worth noting that the results are promising, since the control group showed higher frequency on the last category (the χ^2 test statistic resulted 7.897). On the basis of these good results it was decided to launch phase III trial, provided that the conservative sample size estimate did not exceed $M_{\max} = 500$. A balanced design is, then, applied and the sample size estimates given by the

Table 8.2   Classification of the phase II outcomes of the variable of primary interest in the Treatment and in the Control group of Example 8.2.

	1	2	3	
Treatment	11	43	7	61
	18.03%	70.49%	11.48%	
Control	12	30	19	61
	19.67%	49.18%	31.15%	

PWS, 3QS and 1SES strategies are computed. Under balancing, the link function simplifies in $l(u) = u_1/2$.

In particular, the following estimates of the noncentrality parameter are obtained: $\ell_{61} = 6.872$, $\ell_{61}^{75\%} = 3.665$ and $\ell_{61}^{84.1\%} = 2.456$. Then, the estimate of the noncentrality parameter at m data (i.e. $\ell_{m,61}^{\bullet}$) can be obtained through (5.10). For example, for the PWS with $m = 100$ data we have $\ell_{100,61} = (100/2) \times \ell_{61}/(61/2) = 11.266$.

Hence, once α is set at 5%, the estimates of $SP(m)$ for PWS, 3QS and 1SES are computed and reported in Figure 8.1. Finally, according to (8.3), $M_{61} = 113$, $M_{61}^{75\%} = 211$ and $M_{61}^{84.1\%} = 315$ is obtained (these are the estimated sizes for each group).

8.1.3   Final comments

If the C categories are ordered (for example when $C = 3$, referring to a certain state of illness: mild, moderate and severe), then a test statistic more appropriate than the usual χ^2 test can be adopted. At first, more specific alternative hypotheses should be defined, and then the cumulative chi-square statistic may be applied (see Hirotsu, 1986). Alternatively, exact inference may be applied, by adopting the permutation technique (see, for example, Agresti et al., 1990). In case C is quite large, one can resort to the Wilcoxon rank-sum test (see next Chapter). With all these tests the general nonparametric SP estimation technique that will be introduced in the next Chapter can be applied.

8.2   Test for S couples of binomial distributions: the Mantel-Haenszel test

Stratified categorical data are now considered, with S strata and only two categories. In practice, the outcome is binary (i.e. it belongs to $\{0, 1\}$), and the strata may represent the different centers, experimental sites, or baseline states of illness. The data are, therefore, represented by $X_{s,ij} \in \{0, 1\}$, where $s = 1, \ldots, S$ represents

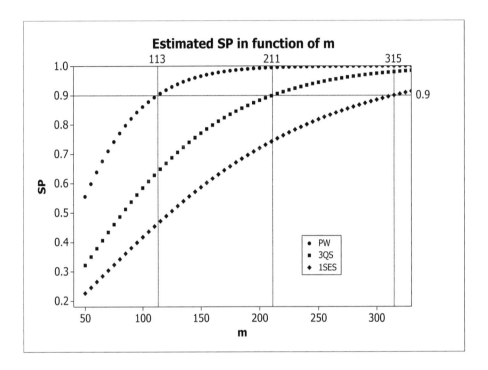

Figure 8.1 *PWS, 3QS and 1SES estimates of SP for balanced designs, based on $n_1 = n_2 = 61$ phase II data of Example 8.2, in function of the phase III sample size m.*

the stratum, $i = 1, 2$ the treatment (group), and $j = 1, \ldots, m_{s,i}$ where $m_{s,i}$ is the sample size of the i-th treatment in the s-th stratum. Moreover, the binary outcome 1, or 0, may represent the success, or failure, of the drug in the single experimental unit/patient.

For each group and stratum there is a specific probability to result in 1, that is, $P(X_{s,ij} = 1) = \pi_{s,i}$, with $s = 1, \ldots, S$, $i = 1, 2$. Here, $_tF_i = \{\pi_{1,i}, \ldots, \pi_{S,i}\}$.

The null hypothesis is that of no difference between $_tF_1$ and $_tF_2$, that is, between the probabilities of the two drugs to result in 1 for every stratum: $H_0 : \pi_{s,1} = \pi_{s,2}$ for every $s = 1, \ldots, S$; the alternative is that there are differences among treatments in at least one stratum: $H_1 : \pi_{s,1} \neq \pi_{s,2}$ for some s.

Now, let's build the test statistic. For every generic stratum s, consider the counts of sample outcomes equal to 1 of the i-th group: $m_{s,i,1} = (\#X_{s,ij} = 1)$. Moreover, let $m_{s,\bullet,1} = m_{s,1,1} + m_{s,2,1}$ the total number of successful outcomes in the s-th stratum, and $m_s = m_{s,1} + m_{s,2}$ the total number of outcomes in the s-th stratum.

The estimator of the probability of success under the null is, for the s-th stratum, $p_{s,\bullet} = m_{s,\bullet,1}/m_s$. Consequently, the estimator of the count of success for the first treatment in the s-th stratum under H_0 is $m_{s,\bullet,1} = p_{s,\bullet}m_{s,1}$.

The test statistic is based on the differences between the observed counts of success of the first group (i.e. $m_{s,1,1}$) and the expected counts under the null ($m_{s,\bullet,1}$). In particular, the square of the sum of the differences is adopted, adequately standardized through the total variance, i.e. the sum of the variances of the S differences. Being v_s the variance of the s-th difference, i.e. $v_s = m_{s,1}m_{s,2}m_{s,\bullet,1}(m_s - m_{s,\bullet,1})/m_s^2(m_s - 1)$, the test statistic is:

$$T_m = \frac{[\sum_{s=1}^{S}(m_{s,1,1} - m_{s,\bullet,1})]^2}{\sum_{s=1}^{S} v_s}$$

Under H_0, T_m is asymptotically (i.e. as m increases) distributed as a χ^2 with 1 degree of freedom. The critical value is, therefore, $t_{m,1-\alpha} = \chi_1^{2^{-1}}(1 - \alpha)$, so that the statistical test (5.1) becomes:

$$\psi_\alpha(T_m) = \begin{cases} 1 & \text{if} \quad T_m > \chi_1^{2^{-1}}(1 - \alpha) \\ 0 & \text{if} \quad T_m \leq \chi_1^{2^{-1}}(1 - \alpha) \end{cases} \tag{8.4}$$

From (5.2) the p-value of this test is $1 - \chi_1^2(T_m)$.

8.2.1 Power and RP estimation

Several approximations for the power of this test have been proposed. Among these are Gail (1973), Berger et al. (1979) and Munoz and Rosner (1984). Then, Wittes and Wallenstein (1987) provided a simple solution based on the approximation of the noncentrality parameter for the distribution of this test statistic. In particular, they gave:

$$_t\lambda_m \approx \frac{(\sum_{s=1}^{S} m_{s,1}m_{s,2}(\pi_{s,1} - \pi_{s,2})/m_s)^2}{\sum_{s=1}^{S} m_{s,1}m_{s,2}(m_{s,1}\pi_{s,1} + m_{s,2}\pi_{s,2})(m_s - m_{s,1}\pi_{s,1} - m_{s,2}\pi_{s,2})/m_s^3} \tag{8.5}$$

The test statistic T_m is therefore approximately distributed as a $\chi_{1,\,_t\lambda_m}^2$, and the approximated power function, being λ_m the generic noncentrality parameter, is:

$$\pi(\alpha, \lambda_m) = 1 - \chi_{1,\lambda_m}^2(\chi_1^{2^{-1}}(1 - \alpha))$$

Table 8.3 Counts of Responders and Non-Responders in the four strata of illness, in the Treatment and in the Control group of Example 8.3.

	NR	R	Tot.
1st str. - Treatment	5 (62.5%)	3 (37.5%)	8
Control	6 (75%)	2 (25%)	8
2nd str. - Treatment	9 (60%)	6 (40%)	15
Control	12 (75%)	4 (25%)	16
3st str. - Treatment	11 (57.9%)	8 (42.1%)	19
Control	12 (60%)	8 (40%)	20
4th str. - Treatment	6 (54.5%)	5 (45.5%)	11
Control	8 (80%)	2 (20%)	10

When a sample of size n is given, the γ lower bound for $_t\lambda_n$ (i.e. ℓ_n^γ) can be computed through the root v of:

$$\chi_{1,v}^2(T_n) = \gamma$$

and the RP estimator results:

$$\hat{RP}_\alpha^\gamma = 1 - \chi_{1,\ell_n^\gamma}^2(\chi_1^{2^{-1}}(1-\alpha))$$

The pointwise RP estimator (i.e. $\hat{RP}_\alpha = \hat{RP}_\alpha^{50\%}$) can be adopted for RP-testing, and the RP-test provides equal results to the test above (8.4).

■ **EXAMPLE 8.3**

A phase III trial regarding the assumption of a certain drug in patients with 4 different states of illness at baseline was conducted to evaluate if the response rate was higher than that given by the placebo. The type I error level α was 5%. 107 patients were allocated with an approximately 50% rate to the two treatment groups in each of the four strata. Regression in illness status was considered a positive response. Table 8.3 reports the count of responders/non-responders (viz. R/NR), showing a slightly higher responder rate in the treatment group.

The sum of differences in the numerator of the test statistic results 3.1998, and that of variances 6.3065, so that the test statistic resulted 1.6234, giving a p-value of $0.2026 = 1 - \chi_1^2(1.6234)$ (see Table A.4) and, finally, a non-significant result. The pointwise RP estimate resulted of 24.26%, according to RP-testing (i.e. lower than $1/2$).

8.2.2 Sample size estimation

In order to derive $\ell^\gamma_{m,n}$ from ℓ^γ_n some assumptions should be made regarding the fixed rates of allocation per stratum and per group in the pilot and in the final experiments. Being n_{tot} and m_{tot} the total sample sizes of phases II and III, respectively (i.e. $n_{tot} = \sum_{s=1}^S n_s$ and $m_{tot} = \sum_{s=1}^S m_s$), let $f_s = n_s/n_{tot} = m_s/m_{tot}$ be the fixed rate of allocation to the s-th stratum, and let $\theta_s = n_{s,1}/n_s = m_{s,1}/m_s$ be the fixed rate of allocation to the treatment group in the s-th stratum. Then, the noncentrality parameter in (8.5) simplifies into:

$$_t\lambda_m \approx \frac{\sqrt{m}_{tot}(\sum_{s=1}^S f_s\theta_s(1 - \theta_s)(\pi_{s,1} - \pi_{s,2}))^2}{\sum_{s=1}^S f_s\theta_s(1 - \theta_s)(\theta_s\pi_{s,1} + (1 - \theta_s)\pi_{s,2})(1 - \theta_s\pi_{s,1} - (1 - \theta_s)\pi_{s,2})}$$

Under these fixed rate conditions it is therefore easy to see that the link function is simply $l(u) = u_{tot} = |u|_1$, and so we have $\ell^\gamma_{m,n} = \ell^\gamma_n m_{tot}/n_{tot}$. Consequently, the conservative sample size estimator is:

$$M^\gamma_n = \min\{m \quad : \quad 1 - \chi^2_{1,\ell^\gamma_{m,n}}(\chi_1^{2^{-1}}(1 - \alpha)) > 1 - \beta\} \qquad (8.6)$$

The effect size is difficult to interpret here, in analogy with the χ^2 test of the previous section (see 8.1.2). Once again, in order to set a launching rule we suggest resorting either to the statistical significance criterion or to the maximum sample size criterion. Also, to compute the OP and to apply COS, the explanation in the last two paragraphs of Section 8.1.2 remains valid.

8.2.3 Final comments

Exact inference can also be applied in this situation, for example, by applying the algorithm proposed by Pagano and Tritchler (1983a). A survey of exact inference for contingency tables was provided by Agresti (1992). For complicated testing situations, where it may be difficult to obtain power approximations and then to estimate the power, such as those based on exact computations, there is the possibility of resorting to the general nonparametric SP estimation technique that will be presented in the next Chapter.

8.3 On chi-square RP estimates

In contrast to the curves of RP estimates given by t-distributions (see Figure 6.3), which for small p-values were higher than those given by Gaussian distribution, those provided by χ^2 distributions are lower. For example, in Figure 8.2 some RP curves were drawn (with $\gamma = 50\%, 90\%, 95\%$) for the χ^2 distribution with 3 dfs, together with the corresponding ones for the Gaussian distribution, already shown in Figure

2.5 ($\alpha = 2.5\%$, one-tailed). It is worth noting that as the dfs increase, the RP estimates of the χ^2 distribution become closer to that of the Gaussian distribution.

Finally, note that the RP estimates reported in Example 8.1 can be extrapolated from Figure 8.2.

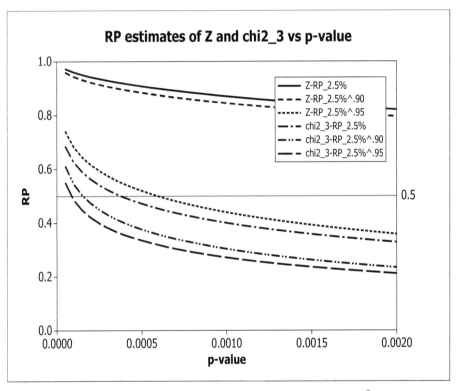

Figure 8.2 *Conservative RP estimates as a function of the p-value for the χ^2-test, in relation with those of the Z-test. The one-tailed setting is considered, with $\alpha = 2.5\%$.*

CHAPTER 9

GENERAL NONPARAMETRIC SP ESTIMATION - WITH APPLICATIONS TO THE WILCOXON TEST

In this Chapter the techniques for estimating the SP through the adoption of a completely nonparametric approach are first developed. They are based on the plug-in of the empirical distribution functions, which are nonparametric estimators of the unknown distributions of the variables of interest. Then, lower bounds for the SP can be obtained thanks to bootstrap techniques.

Applications of SP estimation are provided for one of the most widely used two-sample nonparametric tests, viz. the two-sample Wilcoxon rank-sum test. Moreover, also semi-parametric SP estimation techniques, based on the asymptotic normality of the test statistic, are shown for this test. Applications to RP estimation and testing and to conservative sample size estimation are given, together with numerical examples. It is worth noting that the nonparametric plug-in and bootstrap approach for estimating the SP can be easily applied to other nonparametric tests.

Success Probability Estimation with Applications to Clinical Trials, First Edition.
By Daniele De Martini Copyright © 2013 John Wiley & Sons, Inc.

9.1   The nonparametric model

The general model of the nonparametric framework is, regarding the first part of its definition, analogous to that of the parametric one introduced in Chapter 5. F_1 and F_2 represent the generic distributions of the variables of interest in the new treatment and in the control populations. The couple (F_1, F_2) belongs to $\mathcal{F}$, a family of couples of distributions over $S \subset R \times R$. Then, $\mathcal{F}_0$ is the subset of couples of distributions representing an ineffective new treatment. Now, let $_tF_1$ and $_tF_2$ represent the true distributions of the variables of interest. The hypotheses are $H_0 : (\,_tF_1,\,_tF_2) \in \mathcal{F}_0$, versus the alternative of the effectiveness of the new drug: $H_1 : (\,_tF_1,\,_tF_2) \in \mathcal{F}\backslash\mathcal{F}_0$.

The random variables $X_{i,j}, j = 1, m_i$, are assumed to be independent and identically distributed, with distribution $_tF_i, i = 1, 2$. Once again $m = (m_1, m_2)$, and the whole sample from both populations is $\mathbf{X_m}$.

In this nonparametric setting the shape of $_tF_i$'s is unknown, and consequently the distribution G_m of the test statistic $T_m = \mathcal{T}(\mathbf{X_m}) \in R$ is unknown too. The type I error probability is α, and the Acceptance and Rejection regions are defined as $A_{m,\alpha}$ and $R_{m,\alpha}$, so the statistical test is:

$$\psi_\alpha(T_m) = \begin{cases} 1 & \text{if} \quad T_m \in R_{m,\alpha} \\ 0 & \text{if} \quad T_m \in A_{m,\alpha} \end{cases} \tag{9.1}$$

In some situations the distribution G_m is known under the null, and it is named $G_{m,0}$. To remain within the comparison of two samples, this is the case of the Wilcoxon rank-sum test, the control median test and the Kolmogorov-Smirnov test (see Gibbons and Chakraborti, 2003, Conover, 1999), to name a few. On such occasions, the Acceptance and Rejection regions are usually defined on the basis of the quantiles of $G_{m,0}$. Being $t_{m,1-\alpha} = G_{m,0}^{-1}(1 - \alpha)$ the critical value, the rejection region is often of the form $R_\alpha = (t_{m,1-\alpha}, +\infty)$. For instance, for other tests G_m is not known even under the null, e.g. in permutation tests or in bootstrap tests (see Hoeffding, 1952, Efron and Tibshirani, 2003, Chapters 15 and 16).

The p-value is the type I error probability that should have been defined in order to find the test statistic T_m on the boundary between $A_{m,\alpha}$ and $R_{m,\alpha}$. Given $G_{m,0}$, when $R_\alpha = (t_{m,1-\alpha}, +\infty)$ the p-value results $1 - G_{m,0}^{-1}(T_m)$.

In the general nonparametric situation the power of the test is a functional: it depends, indeed, not only on one argument (in the parametric model the latter was λ) but on the generic distribution functions F_i's. In formulas we have:

$$\pi(\alpha, m, F_1, F_2) = P_{F_1, F_2}(T_m \in R_{m,\alpha}) \tag{9.2}$$

Now, consider $_tF_1$ and $_tF_2$ so that the SP, defined in analogy with (5.4), is:

$$SP = P_{_tF_1,\,_tF_2}(T_m \in R_{m,\alpha}) = P_{_tF_1,\,_tF_2}(\psi_\alpha(T_m) = 1) \tag{9.3}$$

When $R_\alpha = (t_{m,1-\alpha}, +\infty)$ this SP becomes $P_{tF_1, tF_2}(T_m > t_{m,1-\alpha})$.

9.2 General nonparametric SP estimation

When two pilot samples of size n_1 and n_2 are available from $_tF_1$ and $_tF_2$, respectively, the *Empirical Distribution Functions* (edf) $\hat{F}_{1,n_1}$ and $\hat{F}_{2,n_2}$ can be derived. In detail: $\hat{F}_{i,n_i}(t) = \sum_{j=1}^{n_i} I\{X_{i,j} \leq t\}/n_i$, $i = 1, 2$. Then, the latter edfs can be plugged into the power functional (9.2) to obtain the plug-in estimator of the SP in (9.3), which now assumes the name $SP(m)$. Formally, we have:

$$\hat{SP}_n^{PI}(m) = P_{\hat{F}_{1,n_1}, \hat{F}_{2,n_2}}(\psi_\alpha(T_m^*) = 1 \mid \mathbf{X_n}) \tag{9.4}$$

Here above, $n = (n_1, n_2)$ in analogy with m, and T_m^* is defined in analogy with T_m but on the basis of the samples $X_{i,j}^*$, $j = 1, m_i$, drawn from $\hat{F}_{i,n_i}$, $i = 1, 2$ (in other words, $X_{i,j}^*$ are re-sampled from the edfs).

Lower bounds for the SP can be obtained by bootstrapping $\hat{SP}_n^{PI}(m)$. Let $\hat{F}_{1,n_1}^*$ be the empirical distribution function given by a sample of size n_1 drawn from $\hat{F}_{1,n_1}$, and let $\hat{F}_{2,n_2}^*$ be built analogously on the basis of a sample of size n_2 drawn from $\hat{F}_{2,n_2}$. Then, consider the bootstrap estimator of the SP:

$$\hat{SP}_n^{BO}(m) = \pi(\alpha, m, \hat{F}_{1,n_1}^*, \hat{F}_{2,n_2}^*)$$

whose distribution, denoted by:

$$H_{\hat{F}_{1,n_1}, \hat{F}_{2,n_2}}(t) = P_{\hat{F}_{1,n_1}, \hat{F}_{2,n_2}}(\hat{SP}_n^{BO}(m) \leq t \mid \mathbf{X_n}),$$

is known given the pilot samples $\mathbf{X_n}$. A bootstrap γ-lower bound for the SP, namely $\hat{SP}_n^{\gamma;BO}(m)$, is given by the $1 - \gamma$ quantile of $H_{\hat{F}_{1,n_1}, \hat{F}_{2,n_2}}$. Formally, we have:

$$\hat{SP}_n^{\gamma,BO}(m) = H_{\hat{F}_{1,n_1}, \hat{F}_{2,n_2}}^{-1}(1 - \gamma) \tag{9.5}$$

Actually, this bootstrap solution provides just an approximated lower bound, since it is such that:

$$P(\hat{SP}_n^{\gamma,BO}(m) \leq SP(m)) \approx \gamma$$

This signifies that $\hat{SP}_n^{\gamma,BO}(m)$ might not respect the nominal amount of conservativeness γ.

Both plug-in and bootstrap approaches in (9.4) and (9.5), respectively, are consistent: when the pilot sample size $n = (n_1, n_2)$ increases, $\hat{SP}_n^{PI}(m)$ and $\hat{SP}_n^{\gamma,BO}(m)$ tend to $SP(m)$ in (9.3); moreover, the approximation accuracy of the bootstrap lower bound improves, that is, $P(\hat{SP}_n^{\gamma,BO}(m) \leq SP)$ tends to γ.

These theoretical results of consistency come from the possibility of considering $\hat{SP}_n^{PI}(m)$ as a V-statistic of degree m (De Martini, 2011a). For an introduction to V-statistics see Serfling (1980). Since it has been proved that the bootstrap of V-statistics holds (Arcones and Giné, 1992) it is possible to bootstrap $\hat{SP}_n^{PI}(m)$ and to use the quantiles of its bootstrap distribution (i.e. $\hat{SP}_n^{\gamma,BO}(m)$) as statistical lower bounds for $SP(m)$.

Bootstrap performances can be improved in terms of precision by some computationally intensive techniques. In particular, *calibration* (see Efron and Tibshirani, 1993) can be applied to reduce the gap between the nominal and the actual amount of conservativeness of SP estimates, that is, in order to bring $P(\hat{SP}_n^{\gamma,BO}(m) \leq SP(m))$ nearer to γ even at a fixed n. In practice, there exists $c(\gamma)$ such that $P(\hat{SP}_n^{c(\gamma),BO}(m) \leq SP(m)) = \gamma$. In other words, there exists a nominal amount of conservativeness $c(\gamma)$ which, when applied to the lower bound $\hat{SP}_n^{\gamma,BO}(m)$, provides the desired amount of conservativeness γ. Then, $c(\gamma)$ is first estimated by, say $\hat{c}_n(\gamma)$, and subsequently the computed estimate is put in practice, to obtain $\hat{SP}_n^{\hat{c}_n(\gamma),BO}(m)$. For example, this technique resulted very useful for estimating the SP of clinical trials with multiple endpoints (see Lucadamo et al., 2013).

Note that, given the pilot samples $\mathbf{X_n}$, the plug-in estimate $\hat{SP}_n^{PI}(m)$ and the bootstrap lower bound $\hat{SP}_n^{\gamma,BO}(m)$ can be computed exactly. However, the latter computations would be quite heavy and time consuming, so that *Monte Carlo* (MC) approximations are usually adopted. Nevertheless, the precision of these approximations can be controlled by an appropriate setting of the computational parameters, so that in practice they can be considered negligible.

The Bayesian nonparametric estimation of SP can be performed in analogy with the parametric one, in order to then apply CSSE. The bootstrap distribution of $\hat{SP}_n^{PI}(m)$ plays the role of the fiducial distribution of the parametric framework (see Section 5.5). So, in analogy with 3.23:

$$\hat{SP}_n^{Bas;BO}(m) = \int_0^1 \hat{SP}_n^{\gamma;BO}(m)\,d\gamma$$

Finally, it is noteworthy that the general SP estimation technique presented here may be applied to many different tests, which consider one or more samples, in univariate or multivariate situations. For instance, it may be used in all situations cited in Sections 7.1.3, 7.2.3, 8.1.3 and 8.2.3.

9.3   The Wilcoxon rank-sum test

When the distributions of the variables of interest in the populations (i.e. F_1 and F_2) are continuous but not Gaussian, the Wilcoxon rank-sum test (WRS) is usually applied. Sometimes the use of the WRS is planned before analyzing data, whereas on some other occasions experimenters resort to it once a test for the normality of the data (such as the Kolmogorov-Smirnov test, see Gibbons and Chakraborti, 2003) has provided significant results. (In clinical trials, eventual modifications of statistical analysis should be clearly stated in the experimental protocol.)

In general, when the distributions are not Gaussian the WRS is often more sensitive than the t-test, providing higher power (see, for example, Blair and Higgins, 1980) and so higher SP.

The WRS evaluates whether X_1 (treatment) is larger than X_2 (control). To be precise, the WRS concerns the stochastic ordering between X_1 and X_2. If X_1 and X_2 have the same shape (i.e. $F_1(t) = F_2(t - \delta)$), the test evaluates the difference between the medians. Consequently, the statistical hypotheses are $H_0 : {}_tF_1 = {}_tF_2$ vs $H_1 : {}_tF_1(t) \leq {}_tF_2(t) \,\forall t$, and ${}_tF_1(t) < {}_tF_2(t)$ for some t.

The test statistic T_m counts how many data of the first sample are higher than those of the second one. So, the test statistic turns out to be:

$$T_m = \sum_{i=1}^{m_1} \sum_{j=1}^{m_2} I_{ij} \,, \qquad \text{where} \qquad I_{ij} = \begin{cases} 1 & \text{if } X_{1,i} > X_{2,j} \\ 0 & \text{otherwise} \end{cases}.$$

The greater the value of T_m, the stronger the empirical evidence against H_0. The latter hypothesis is, therefore, rejected for large values of T_m. Under the null, the distribution G_m of T_m (i.e. $G_{m,0}$) is known and it does not depend on ${}_tF_1$ and ${}_tF_2$. For this reason WRS is a *distribution free* test. Then, being $w_{m,1-\alpha}$ the $(1 - \alpha)$-quantile of $G_{m,0}$, the rejection region is $R_{m,\alpha} = (w_{m,1-\alpha}, \infty)$ and the WRS test, according to (9.1), is:

$$\psi_\alpha(T_m) = \begin{cases} 1 & \text{if } \quad T_m > w_{m,1-\alpha} \\ 0 & \text{if } \quad T_m \leq w_{m,1-\alpha} \end{cases} \tag{9.6}$$

The critical value of the test, i.e. $w_{m,1-\alpha}$, can be calculated iteratively, for example, resorting to Gibbons and Chakraborti (2003), Chapter 6; for faster computations see, for example, Pagano and Tritchler (1983b). The name "rank-sum test" comes from the possibility of obtaining the statistic T_m through the sum of the ranks of the first sample data in the overall set of data (for further details see, for example, Lehmann, 1975).

It is noteworthy that the test statistic T_m is related to the random event "X_1 greater than X_2"; actually T_m counts these kind of events among the two samples. Defining ${}_tp_1 = P_{{}_tF_1, {}_tF_2}(X_1 > X_2)$, then T_m/m_1m_2 is the empirical frequency of the event above, and so it is also an estimator of ${}_tp_1$. Under the null, ${}_tp_1 = 1/2$, where ${}_tp_1 > 1/2$ under the alternative. Nevertheless, it is not correct to write the statistical hypotheses in terms of ${}_tp_1$. Indeed, ${}_tp_1 = 1/2$ does not imply H_0, and $G_{m,0}$ is derived under ${}_tF_1 = {}_tF_2$ and not under the former assumption.

Table 9.1   Relationship between p_1 and δ under the location shift model.

p_1	Amplitude of the effect size δ		
	Uniform	Normal	Bi-expon.
0.5	0.0	0.0	0.0
0.55	0.1778	0.1777	0.1423
0.6	0.3657	0.3583	0.2895
0.65	0.5658	0.5449	0.4461
0.7	0.7808	0.7416	0.6173
0.75	1.0146	0.9539	0.8104

$_tp_1$ is often viewed as the nonparametric effect size (see, for example, Newcombe, 2006a). Since $_tp_1$ varies on a different scale with respect to the effect size $\delta_t = (\mu_1 - \mu_2)/\sigma$ adopted when the distributions are Gaussian, it might be useful to make $_tp_1$ and δ_t comparable, for instance, to set thresholds of clinical relevance. To this aim Table 9.1 reports the values of the generic δ in function of some values of the generic $p_1 = P_{F_1,F_2}(X_1 > X_2)$, for some distributions with unitary variance under the location shift model (i.e. F_1 and F_2 have equal shape and are different in location: $F_1(t) = F_2(t - \delta)$).

9.3.1   Power, SP and their approximations

Under the alternative hypothesis the distribution G_m depends on the whole distribution functions F_1 and F_2. Then, according to (9.2), the power is the following *functional*:

$$\pi(\alpha, m, F_1, F_2) = P_{F_1,F_2}(T_m > w_{m,1-\alpha}) \tag{9.7}$$

and the SP in (9.3) becomes:

$$SP(m) = P_{_tF_1,\,_tF_2}(T_m > w_{m,1-\alpha}) \tag{9.8}$$

The functional in (9.7) can be calculated by resorting to computationally intensive algorithms, e.g. the Monte Carlo method. Other possible approximations of it are based on the asymptotic distribution of T_m, i.e. the asymptotic shape of G_m, whose behavior is normal (see Lehmann, 1975).

The standardized version of the generic T_m, i.e. $(T_m - m_1m_2p_1)/\sqrt{Var(T_m)}$, tends to the standard normal as m increases. The variance of T_m depends on p_1 and it is also a function of two other parameters regarding the stochastic ordering between F_1 and F_2, which are $p_2 = P_{F_1,F_2}(X_1 > X_2$ and $X_1 > X_2')$ and $p_3 = P_{F_1,F_2}(X_1 >$

X_2 and $X_1' > X_2$), where X_1' and X_1 are independent, and so are X_2' and X_2. In particular:

$$Var(T_m) =$$

$$m_1 m_2 p_1 (1 - p_1) + m_1 m_2 (m_2 - 1)(p_2 - p_1^2) + m_1 m_2 (m_1 - 1)(p_3 - p_1^2) \quad (9.9)$$

Exploiting the fact that under the null $p_1 = 1/2$ and $p_2 = p_3 = 1/3$, through simple algebra the following approximation for the power functional (9.7) can be derived:

$$\pi(\alpha, m, F_1, F_2) \approx \pi^{Le}(\alpha, m, F_1, F_2)$$

$$= \Phi\left(\frac{m_1 m_2 (p_1 - 1/2) - z_{1-\alpha}\sqrt{m_1 m_2 (m_1 + m_2 + 1)/12}}{\sqrt{Var(T_m)}}\right) \quad (9.10)$$

where Le stands for Lehmann. Moreover, Noether (1987) suggested an easier approximation based on the above formula and on the assumption that when F_1 and F_2 are quite close to each other, $Var(T_m)$ is well approximated by its value under the null, that is:

$$Var_0(T_m) = m_1 m_2 (m_1 + m_2 + 1)/12$$

It is therefore easy to obtain the following approximation, where No stands for Noether:

$$\pi(\alpha, m, F_1, F_2) \approx \pi^{No}(\alpha, m, F_1, F_2)$$

$$= \Phi(\sqrt{12 m_1 m_2 / (m_1 + m_2 + 1)}(p_1 - 1/2) - z_{1-\alpha}) \quad (9.11)$$

Note that these approximations of the power (9.7) are no more a functional, but simply a function of p_i's. This allows the performance of SP estimation using semiparametric techniques, as will be shown in the next Subsection.

Defining with $_t p_i$ the true value of p_i, $i = 2, 3$, that come from $_t F_1$ and $_t F_2$, and being $_t Var(T_m)$ the true variance obtained by plugging the $_t p_i$'s into (9.9), the approximations of the SP obtained from Lehmann's and Noether's power approximations are:

$$SP^{Le}(m) = \Phi\left(\frac{m_1 m_2 (_t p_1 - 1/2) - z_{1-\alpha}\sqrt{m_1 m_2 (m_1 + m_2 + 1)/12}}{\sqrt{_t Var(T_m)}}\right) \quad (9.12)$$

and

$$SP^{No}(m) = \Phi(\sqrt{12 m_1 m_2 / (m_1 + m_2 + 1)}(_t p_1 - 1/2) - z_{1-\alpha}) \quad (9.13)$$

As m increases, $SP^{Le}(m)$ and $SP^{No}(m)$ tend to the true $SP(m)$ in (9.8).

9.3.2 SP estimation

In order to estimate the SP, assume now that a pilot sample of size n_i from $_t F_i$ is available, $i = 1, 2$.

Exact SP estimation can be performed, either pointwise or conservatively, through the nonparametric estimators (9.4) and (9.5) introduced in Section 9.2. This means that these estimators tend to the exact SP in (9.8). In this way, SP estimation is consistent but it is computationally heavy. When $\gamma = 50\%$, $\hat{SP}_n^{50\%,BO}(m) \approx \hat{SP}_n^{PI}(m)$, so that the latter estimator may be considered one of the family of the former.

The approximated estimation of the SP is based on power approximations (9.10) and (9.11). Let us first define the natural estimators of p_i's, that are:

$$\hat{p}_{1,n} = T_n / n_1 n_2$$

$$\hat{p}_{2,n} = \sum_{i=1}^{n_1} \sum_{j=1}^{n_2} \sum_{k=1}^{n_2} I_{ij} I_{ik} / n_1 n_2^2$$

and

$$\hat{p}_{3,n} = \sum_{i=1}^{n_1} \sum_{j=1}^{n_1} \sum_{k=1}^{n_2} I_{ik} I_{jk} / n_1^2 n_2$$

Then, plugging these estimators into (9.10) and (9.11), two SP estimators based on asymptotic normality (AN) of G_m are derived, namely $\hat{SP}_n^{Le}(m)$ and $\hat{SP}_n^{No}(m)$, respectively. These can be considered semiparametric estimators (see also Wang et al., 2003).

To compute lower bounds for the SP by exploiting the AN of G_m, confidence intervals for the $_t p_i$'s should be computed. Nevertheless, the SP depends mainly on $_t p_1$, whereas $_t p_2$ and $_t p_3$ are nuisance parameters regarding the variability of T_m only. So, AN lower bounds can be obtained through confidence intervals for $_t p_1$ and pointwise estimates of $_t p_2$ and $_t p_3$.

There are various methods for computing confidence intervals for $_t p_1$, as widely illustrated by Newcombe (2006b). In particular, this author suggests the method based on the following equation in v, where $n^* = (n_1 + n_2)/2 - 1$:

$$|\hat{p}_{1,n} - v| = z_\gamma \sqrt{\frac{v(1-v)[1 + n^*(1-v)/(2-v) + n^* v/(1+v)]}{n_1 n_2}} \tag{9.14}$$

The smallest root of this equation is an approximated γ-lower bound for $_t p_1$, namely $\hat{p}_{1,n}^\gamma$. This solution has no closed form and it may be computed iteratively. Finally the AN based lower bounds are derived by plugging $\hat{p}_{1,n}^\gamma$, $\hat{p}_{2,n}$ and $\hat{p}_{3,n}$ into (9.10) and (9.11), obtaining $\hat{SP}_n^{\gamma,Le}(m)$ and $\hat{SP}_n^{\gamma,No}(m)$, respectively. It is easy to see that when $\gamma = 50\%$ the above equation gives $\hat{p}_{1,n}^{50\%} = \hat{p}_{1,n}$, so that 50% conservative AN estimators of the SP coincide with pointwise ones.

It should be noted that when the size of the pilot samples n diverges $\hat{SP}_n^{Le}(m)$ and $\hat{SP}_n^{\gamma,Le}(m)$, $\hat{SP}_n^{No}(m)$ and $\hat{SP}_n^{\gamma,No}(m)$ do not tend to the exact SP in (9.8), but to their respective SP approximations (9.12) and (9.13). These AN based estimators are, therefore, not consistent. Moreover, when n increases, the lower bounds $\hat{SP}_n^{\gamma,Le}(m)$ and $\hat{SP}_n^{\gamma,No}(m)$, which are approximated ones like the bootstrap solution in (9.5), improve their accuracy with respect to their approximated SP and not to the exact SP. In other words, considering, for example, the Lehmann lower bound, it follows that $P(\hat{SP}_n^{\gamma,Le}(m) \leq SP^{Le}(m))$ tends to γ, where $P(\hat{SP}_n^{\gamma,Le}(m) \leq SP(m))$ does not (actually, this probability tends either to 0 or to 1, since $SP^{Le}(m)$ is either higher or lower than $SP(m)$).

Nevertheless, the gap between the exact SP and the approximated ones, i.e. the structural bias, decreases as the sample size m increases. Further explanations can be found in De Martini (2011a), Section 3.3.

A wide simulation study has been conducted in order to evaluate which family of conservative SP estimators is the most affordable, among $\hat{SP}_n^{\gamma,Le}(m)$, $\hat{SP}_n^{\gamma,No}(m)$ and $\hat{SP}_n^{\gamma,BO}(m)$, with γ ranging from 50% to 90%; also, several distributions have been adopted for $_tF_1$ and $_tF_2$. The evaluation of results concerned both the departures from γ of the coverage accuracy of the lower bounds and the variability of SP estimators around $SP(m)$. The study showed that when $1 - \beta = 90\%$ and $n \approx M_I \pm M_I/3$, i.e. the operating conditions for CSSE (see Chapter 3), $\hat{SP}_n^{\gamma,BO}(m)$ is the best performer, with a gain of about 49% and 29% with respect to Lehmann's and Noether's approaches, respectively (De Martini, 2011a, Section 3.4). However, AN based estimates can be quickly computed and can therefore be easily applied.

The better performances of $\hat{SP}_n^{\gamma,BO}(m)$ result from the fact that it is a consistent estimator, and that, since the power functional of a nonparametric test depends on the whole distribution functions F_i's, it exploits all the available information (i.e., the empirical distribution functions $\hat{F}_i$'s), not just some distributional parameters as AN techniques do.

9.3.2.1 *Improving bootstrap SP estimation*

Bootstrap estimation may be improved in many ways. Besides calibration, bootstrap-t intervals or BCA intervals can be applied (see Efron and Tibshirani, 1993). A simple technique for improving bootstrap SP estimation for the WRS test consists in replicating and averaging the MC approximations of the SP estimates in (9.4) and (9.5) (De Martini, 2011a, Section 3.5). In practice, R MC approximations of $\hat{SP}_n^{\gamma,BO}(m)$ are computed and their average, namely $\hat{SP}_n^{\gamma,BO,R}(m)$, is adopted for estimating $SP(m)$. The gain in precision with respect to simple bootstrap is about 15% with $R = 10$.

Note that replications also reduce the variability within different MC based bootstrap estimates, which is one of the practical problems of MC-bootstrap.

9.3.3 RP estimation and testing

As explained in Section 2.2, when $n = m$ the SP assumes the meaning of RP. Then, the SP estimators $\hat{SP}_n^\bullet(n)$ (where $\bullet$ stands for PI, Le and No) are denoted here by $\hat{RP}_\alpha^\bullet$. Hence, the test based on RP estimator, in accordance with (2.4), is:

$$\psi_\alpha'(\hat{RP}_\alpha^\bullet) = \begin{cases} 1 & \text{if} \quad \hat{RP}_\alpha^\bullet > 1/2 \\ 0 & \text{if} \quad \hat{RP}_\alpha^\bullet \leq 1/2 \end{cases} \tag{9.15}$$

The RP-based test is denoted here by ψ_α' instead of, just, ψ_α since the outcomes of the former can, in practice, differ from those of the latter, defined in (9.6). Indeed, in order to perform exact RP-testing for this nonparametric test, it is necessary to know the shapes of $_tF_1$ and $_tF_2$. If the shape of $_tF_1$ is given and the model of stochastic ordering under the alternative hypothesis is known (e.g. the location shift model holds), then the two tests would provide equal outcomes, i.e. $\psi_\alpha' = \psi_\alpha$ (De Capitani and De Martini, 2011). However, in practice the distribution shapes are missing, and that's actually the reason why the Wilcoxon test is applied.

Nevertheless, the rate of disagreement between ψ_α' and ψ_α is very small: from 1% or less with small sample sizes (e.g. $n_1 = n_2 = 20$) to 0.1%, and even 0.01%, with large samples (e.g. $n_1 = n_2 = 200$) (see De Capitani and De Martini, 2012).

In practice, RP-testing for the Wilcoxon rank-sum test can be performed only approximately. Remarkably, a disagreement can occur when the test statistic is very close to the boundary of the acceptance/rejection regions, that is, in case T_n is close to $w_{n,1-\alpha}$. For instance, when RP estimates are high there is no disagreement between the classical test and the RP-based one. This implies that checking for RP-based stability criteria in order to evaluate whether outcomes from a single study are strong enough to support effectiveness, according to Section 2.5, is still possible.

For high RP values, i.e. those more interesting for stability evaluations, the nonparametric plug-in estimator $\hat{RP}_\alpha^{PI}$ provides more precise results than the AN based estimators, as shown in De Capitani and De Martini (2012), and is therefore recommended when G-stability is looked at. Favorable results of nonparametric γ-conservative bootstrap estimators in presence of high power are also found in De Martini (2011a), and $\hat{RP}_\alpha^{\gamma,BO}$ is therefore recommended for γ-stability evaluations.

■ **EXAMPLE 9.1**

A phase III trial was conducted in order to evaluate if a certain drug plus a concomitant treatment performed better than the drug alone. The time to progression of illness was considered as the variable of interest and two samples of patients of size $34 = n_1 = n_2$ were recruited. The one-tailed WRS testing (9.6) was adopted for comparing the outcomes of the two groups, and the type I error probability α was set at 2.5%. Then, according to Table A.5, the critical value *of the test was $w_{34,97.5\%} = 737$. A significant difference was observed in favor of the arm under drug plus additional treatment: $T_{34} = 813$ was computed, giving a p-value of 0.2% (it is easy to verify from Table A.5 that T_{34} lies between 786 and 826, which are the critical values with $\alpha = 0.5\%$ and $\alpha = 0.1\%$, so that the p-value results between 0.1% and 0.5%); α^2 is 0.0625% and, since the p-value is higher than this threshold, α^2-stability was not fulfilled. A quick estimate of the RP is obtained by referring to Noether's approximation (9.11). The pointwise estimate of $_tp_1$ resulted $T_{34}/34^2 = \hat{p}_{1,34} = 813/1156 = 70.33\%$, giving an RP estimate of $\hat{RP}_{2.5\%}^{No} = 82.7\%$; G-stability was, therefore, not fulfilled either. The 90%-lower bound for $_tp_1$, obtained through (9.14), resulted $\hat{p}_{1,n}^{90\%} = 61.59\%$, giving the RP conservative estimate $\hat{RP}_{2.5\%}^{90\%,No} = 38.0\%$; neither was 90%-stability obtained, in agreement with both previous criteria. Nonparametric estimators gave $\hat{RP}_{2.5\%}^{PI} = 82.8\%$ and $\hat{RP}_{2.5\%}^{90\%,BO} = 38.2\%$, which are quite close to AN estimates, but this is not always the case.*

9.3.4 Sample size estimation

In accordance with Section 3.1 there exists an ideal sample size M_I, that is, $\min\{m$ such that $SP(m) > 1 - \beta\}$ and the SP is that defined in (9.8).

In order to estimate this M_I, SP estimators should be adopted in analogy with formula (3.2). Given the power to attain $1 - \beta$, the generical conservative sample size estimator is:

$$M_n^{\gamma,\bullet} = \min\{m \quad \text{such that} \quad \hat{SP}_n^{\gamma,\bullet}(m) > 1 - \beta\} \tag{9.16}$$

where $\bullet$ stands for BO, Le and No. As a consequence of the better performances of $\hat{SP}_n^{\gamma,BO}(m)$ for estimating SP with respect to estimators based on AN (some numbers are given in Section 9.3.2), the adoption of $M_n^{\gamma,BO}$ is suggested (see also De Martini, 2011a).

When $\gamma = 50\%$, the bootstrap conservative estimator $M_n^{50\%,BO}$ has a very similar behavior to that of the PWS one, i.e. M_n^{PI}. Computationally, the latter is less heavy. With both estimators the probability to build an underpowered experiment is approximately 50%. The sample size estimators of the conservative strategies 3QS and of 1SES are given, in this nonparametric context, by $M_n^{75\%,BO}$ and $M_n^{84.1\%,BO}$. When replications are used (see Section 9.3.2.1), the γ-conservative bootstrap estimator becomes $M_n^{\gamma,BO,R}$.

For quick sample size estimation the Noether's solution is preferred to Lehmann's one. The estimator for the sample size of the first group, i.e. $M_{I,1}$, is therefore:

$$M_{n,1}^{\gamma,No} \approx \lfloor (1+c)(z_{1-\alpha} + z_{1-\beta})^2/12c(\hat{p}_{1,n}^\gamma - 1/2)^2 \rfloor + 1$$

where $c = m_2/m_1$. In general, $M_n^{\gamma,No}$, besides being less precise than $M_n^{\gamma,BO}$, tends to be overconservative, and consequently it often results larger than the latter. For instance, when $_tF_i$'s are uniform distributions and $M_I = 60$, the differences between $M_{60}^{\gamma,No}$ and $M_{60}^{\gamma,BO}$ vary from -1 to 5 for pointwise estimation, and from -3 to 10 with $\gamma = 80\%$ (De Martini, 2011a). Since $M_I = 60$, these differences are not negligible.

To apply the launching criterion based on the clinical relevance of the effect size $_tp_1$, one should refer to Table 9.1 in order to relate p_1 to δ for setting the launching threshold $p_{1,0L}$. The other two criteria of Section 3.3 may also be adopted, and that based on the maximum sample size is suggested here.

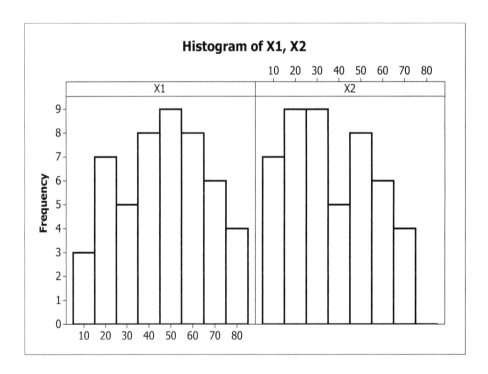

Figure 9.1 *Histograms of the $n_1 = 48$ and $n_2 = 50$ phase II data of Example 9.2.*

■ **EXAMPLE 9.2**

A new drug has been developed to treat a certain disturbance, and the effect must be proved on a score scale. The score increases if the treatment is effective,

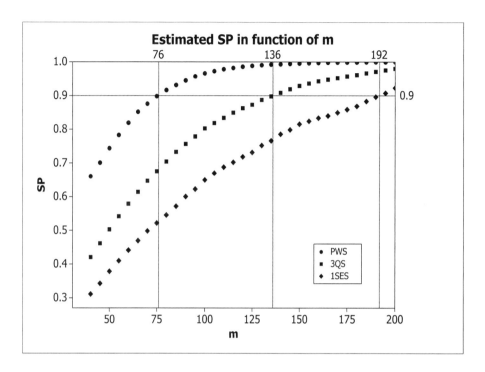

Figure 9.2   *PWS, 3QS and 1SES SP estimates, based on $n_1 = 48$ and $n_2 = 50$ phase II data of Example 9.2, in function of the phase III sample size m.*

and the post-pre differences are considered for the statistical evaluation. These differences are named X_1 and X_2 in the control and in the treatment group, respectively. $n_1 = 48$ and $n_2 = 50$ phase II data were collected, and the experiment showed that the new drug performed well with respect to the control group: the X_1 sample was higher than the X_2 one. In particular, the quartiles of X_1 were 26.6, 48.9 and 63.6, and those of X_2 resulted 21.1, 33.8, 51.2. It is worth noting that the empirical distributions presented a non-Gaussian shape – in Figure 9.1 the histograms of the two groups are reported. Being these results considered promising, the phase III study has to be planned for the one-tailed WRS with $\alpha = 2.5\%$ and $1 - \beta = 90\%$, and is launched provided that the estimated sample size is not greater than $M_{\max} = 500$. A balanced design (i.e. $M_{I,1} = M_{I,2} = M_I$) is adopted and the nonparametric bootstrap estimator of $SP(m)$ in (9.5) is used for estimating M_I. MC approximations are applied in the computation, and $R = 10$ replications (according to 9.3.2.1) are performed *and averaged. SP estimates for the PWS, 3QS and 1SES strategies, in function of the increasing phase III sample size m, are reported in Figure 9.2. For each group, PWS gives $M^{BO,10}_{(48,50)} = 76$, and the sample size estimators of the 3QS and the 1SES strategies give $M^{75\%,BO,10}_{(48,50)} = 136$ and $M^{84.1\%,BO,10}_{(48,50)} = 192$.*

Concerning different CSSE strategies (e.g. PWS, 1SES, ...), they still present different features (i.e. different probabilities to launch, different distributions of sample size estimators, different Average Power, ...), and this is in accordance with the contents of Section 3.4. Exact analytical forms of the quantities of interest, like those in (3.14) or (3.16), cannot be derived since they depend on the $_tF_i$'s shapes, which are unknown. Nevertheless, these quantities can be estimated, in order to then apply the COS strategy. For instance, estimates of the distribution of sample size estimators are shown below.

▣ EXAMPLE 9.3

In Figure 9.3 the estimated distributions of $M^{50\%,BO}_{48,50}$ and $M^{84.1\%,BO}_{48,50}$ (i.e. the bootstrap sample size estimators of PWS and 1SES strategies with the balanced design), conditioned to be lower than 500 and obtained on the basis of the $n = (48,50)$ data of Example 9.2, are shown ($\alpha = 2.5\%$ and $1 - \beta = 90\%$ as in Example 9.2). Formally, these are the distributions of $M^{*;\gamma,BO}_{48,50}$ with $\gamma = 50\%, 84.1\%$, which can be defined in complete analogy to $M^{\gamma,BO}_n$ in (9.16), but it is based on $\hat{F}^*_{i,n_i}$'s (defined in Section 9.2) instead of on $\hat{F}_{i,n_i}$'s, as $M^{\gamma,BO}_n$ is. Note that these two distributions are similar to the analogous ones obtained in the parametric context and reported in Figure 3.2 (see Section 3.4).

Besides the distribution of sample size estimators of the different strategies, their different OPs are also of interest, and are still defined by equation (3.12). An OP formulation like that in (3.17) cannot be obtained since the launch probability, the distribution of $M^{\bullet}_n$ and SP depend on the unknown shapes of the $_tF_i$'s. Nevertheless, the OP can be estimated, and this is what is needed to apply COS.

To apply the launching criterion based on the clinical relevance of the effect size p_1, one should refer to Table 9.1 in order to relate p_1 to δ. Here, the launching rule based on the maximum sample size is adopted.

▣ EXAMPLE 9.4

Continuing Example 9.3. When the maximum sample size is $M_{\max} = 500$, the estimated probability to launch PWS and 1SES are $P_{\hat{F}_{1,48},\hat{F}_{2,50}}(M^{BO}_n \leq 500) = 96.4\%$ and $P_{\hat{F}_{1,48},\hat{F}_{2,50}}(M_n^{.841,BO} \leq 500) = 76.8\%$. In order to estimate the OP, the pointwise estimate of the SP should also be used, and this is $\hat{SP}^{BO}_{48,50}$ reported in Figure 9.2 (the highest function). Through this information

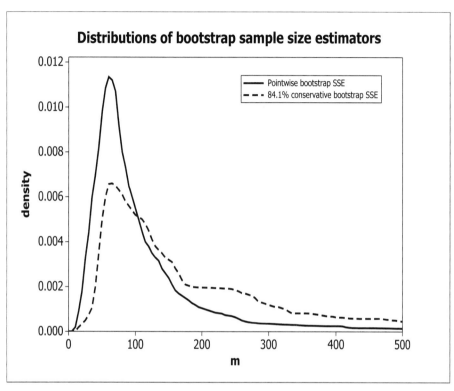

Figure 9.3 *Estimated distributions of nonparametric PWS and 1SES sample size estimators, based on $n_1 = 48$ and $n_2 = 50$ phase II data of Example 9.2.*

$OP_{48,50}(50\%)$ *and* $OP_{48,50}(84.1\%)$ *can be estimated, and their estimates result* 79.8% *and* 71.1%, *respectively.*

To apply the COS strategy, $OP_n(\gamma)$ should be estimated for each $\gamma \in (0,1)$, or at least for γs lying in a sufficiently large set, in order to then find the optimal amount of conservativeness g_n^O to be applied in CSSE.

■ EXAMPLE 9.5

On the basis of the $n = (48, 50)$ phase II data of Example 9.2, for γ ranging from 10% to 90% (with step 1%) $OP_{(48,50)}(\gamma)$ has been estimated for the balanced design (once again $\alpha = 2.5\%$ $1 - \beta = 90\%$). These OP values have been obtained through the combination of: a) the estimated distribution of $M_{(48,50)}^{\gamma,BO,3}$ (i.e. with 3 replications of the MC approximation of $\hat{SP}_{(48,50)}^{\gamma,BO}(m)$); b) *the estimate of the probability to launch, that is,* $P_{\hat{F}_{1,48}, \hat{F}_{2,50}}(M_{(48,50)}^{\gamma, BO, 3} \leq 500)$;

c) the estimated $SP(m)$, *i.e.* $\hat{SP}_{(48,50)}^{BO}(m)$. *The estimates so obtained (i.e.* $\hat{OP}_{(48,50)}(\gamma)$) *are drawn in Figure 9.4, where it is shown that the maximum OP is obtained with* $g_{(48,50)}^{O} = 57\%$, *resulting* 80.2% *(i.e.* $\hat{OP}_{(48,50)}(57\%) = 80.2\%$). *Therefore, COS suggests adopting the* 57%-*conservative sample size estimate, and the bootstrap estimator with* $R = 10$ *(i.e.* $M_{(48,50)}^{57\%, BO, 10}$) *gives* 87 *data per group: this is the nonparametric COS estimated sample size.*

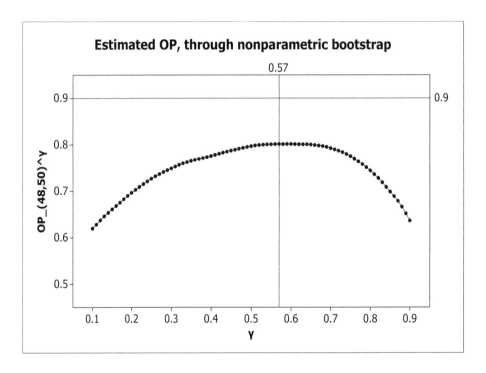

Figure 9.4   *Bootstrap estimated OP, on the basis of the* $n_1 = 48$ *and* $n_2 = 50$ *phase II data of Example 9.2.*

9.3.5   Corrections in sample size estimation

When different distributions occur in phases II and III, it is also possible to correct the bias in sample size estimation in this nonparametric context, in analogy with the techniques shown in Chapter 4. If the difference between the distributions of the two drugs under study in phase III is a certain percentage (i.e. k) of that of the phase II, then a correction k_c can be postulated to be applied in sample size estimation.

Since nonparametric techniques are adopted, instead of applying k_c to the estimator of the effect size (i.e. to use $d^{\bullet}_{II,n} \times k_c$, see Section 4.3.1) the two empirical distributions given by phase II data should be brought closer by the factor k_c. This can be done in different ways, depending on the assumptions made on the model generating the data.

When $_tF_1$ and $_tF_2$ have the same distribution and different location (e.g. $_tF_i$ are uniform on $[\eta_i - a, \eta_i + a]$, $a > 0$, $i = 1, 2$, with $\eta_1 > \eta_2 > 0$), the correction should be applied by subtracting a certain quantity depending on k_c (say, l_c) from the data generated by the larger distribution (i.e. the n_1 data from $_tF_1$). This quantity might be the difference between the medians times the correction, i.e. $l_c = (Med_{1,n_1} - Med_{2,n_2}) \times k_c$. A more sophisticated and robust solution consists in the adoption of the Hodges-Lehmann estimator of the difference between $_tF_i$'s, that is, the median of the $n_1 \times n_2$ differences between the data of the two groups: $HL_n = Med_{i=1,n_1;j=1,n_2}\{X_{1,i} - X_{2,j}\}$; then, $l_c = HL_n \times k_c$.

Therefore, the *corrected* empirical distribution of the first group is $_c\hat{F}_{1,n_1}(t) = \sum_{j=1}^{n_1} I\{X_{1,j} - l_c \le t\}/n_1 = \hat{F}_{1,n_1}(t + l_c)$. Consequently, the sample size can be estimated by adopting $_c\hat{F}_{1,n_1}$ and $\hat{F}_{2,n_2}$ either to compute the nonparametric SP estimator in (9.5), or to compute $\hat{p}_{1,n}$ and its subsequent conservative version through (9.14) to be plugged into AN power approximations.

9.3.6 Discrete distributions

Often, the Wilcoxon rank-sum test is adopted even when the variable of interest is discrete, for example, when a score is being studied. The C different possible outcomes can be defined as U_h, with $h = 1, \ldots, C$, that is, $X_i \in \{U_1, \ldots, U_C\}$, $i = 1, 2$.

In this case the *ties*, i.e. the events $X_{1,i} = X_{2,j}$, for some i and j, can occur and should be taken into account. The test statistic should therefore be modified and one of the possible solutions adopts the so-called *mid-ranks*, that is:

$$T_m = \sum_{i=1}^{m_1} \sum_{j=1}^{m_2} I_{ij} \ , \qquad \text{where} \qquad I_{ij} = \begin{cases} 1 & \text{if } X_{1,i} > X_{2,j} \\ 0.5 & \text{if } X_{1,i} = X_{2,j} \\ 0 & \text{otherwise} \end{cases}$$

Also, $_tp_1$ becomes $P_{_tF_1, _tF_2}(X_1 > X_2) + P(X_1 = X_2)/2$, and it is still estimated by T_m/m_1m_2. The AN of T_m holds: whereas its mean remains the same (i.e. $_tp_1m_1m_2$), the asymptotic variance changes accounting for the number and the frequencies of different ties (see, for example, Lehmann, 1975). In order to provide the Noether's SP estimator, the variance under the null should be derived, and it results

(Gibbons and Chakraborti, 2003, Chapter 6):

$$Var_0(T_m) = \frac{m_1 m_2 (m_1 + m_2 + 1)}{12}$$

$$\times \left(1 - \frac{\sum_{h=1}^{C} [(m_{1,h} + m_{2,h})^3 - m_{1,h} - m_{2,h}]}{(m_1 + m_2)((m_1 + m_2)^2 - 1)} \right)$$

where the notation introduced in Section 8.1 for the $2 \times C$ contingency table has been adopted (i.e. $m_{i,h} = (\#X_{i,j} = U_h)$). Then, in analogy with the Noether SP approximation (9.13), and with its related estimator $\hat{SP}^{\gamma, No}(m)$, the SP estimator accounting for *Ties* is:

$$\hat{SP}^{\gamma, NoT}(m) = \Phi((\hat{p}_{1,n}^{\gamma} - 1/2)/\sqrt{Var_0(T_m)} - z_{1-\alpha})$$

The nonparametric bootstrap estimator $\hat{SP}^{\gamma, BO}(m)$ in (9.5) can still be used, but it should be slightly modified for ties. In practice, the edfs $\hat{F}_{i,n_i}$, $i = 1, 2$, should be smoothed, that is, they should be transformed into continuous functions, in order to avoid too many ties due to re-sampling during MC computations.

Several smoothing techniques are available (see, for example, Silverman, 1986), and these are often based on the concept that a continuous distribution of probability mass $1/n_i$ (named *kernel*) is put around $X_{i,j}$. Other smoothing approaches for the bootstrap can be found in De Martini (2000).

In order to compute $\hat{SP}^{\gamma, BO}(m)$, the sample elements drawn from $\hat{F}_{i,n_i}$ should be affected by a random small variability. For example, a random error $\epsilon_{i,j}$ with mean 0 and small variance may be added to $X_{i,j}$, giving $X_{i,j}^* = X_{i,j} + \epsilon_{i,j}$ used for computing $\hat{F}_{i,n_i}^*$, $i = 1, 2$.

APPENDIX A
TABLES OF QUANTILES

Table A.1: Values of the cdf of the Standard Gaussian, to obtain the critical values of the Z-test.

Table A.2 and A.3: Critical values of the t-test.

Table A.4: Critical values of the χ^2-test.

Tables A.5 and A.6: Critical values of the Wilcoxon test, with $m_1 = m_2$, 120 being the maximum of $m_1 + m_2$.

Table A.7: Critical values of the Wilcoxon test, with sample size rate $k = m_i/m_j = 2$, $i \neq j$, 120 being the maximum of $m_1 + m_2$.

Success Probability Estimation with Applications to Clinical Trials, First Edition.
By Daniele De Martini Copyright © 2013 John Wiley & Sons, Inc.

Table A.1 Values of the cdf of the Standard Gaussian: $\Phi(x)$.

x	0.00	0.01	0.02	0.03	0.04	0.05	0.06	0.07	0.08	0.09
0.0	.5000	.5040	.5080	.5120	.5160	.5199	.5239	.5279	.5319	.5359
0.1	.5398	.5438	.5478	.5517	.5557	.5596	.5636	.5675	.5714	.5753
0.2	.5793	.5832	.5871	.5910	.5948	.5987	.6026	.6064	.6103	.6141
0.3	.6179	.6217	.6255	.6293	.6331	.6368	.6406	.6443	.6480	.6517
0.4	.6554	.6591	.6628	.6664	.6700	.6736	.6772	.6808	.6844	.6879
0.5	.6915	.6950	.6985	.7019	.7054	.7088	.7123	.7157	.7190	.7224
0.6	.7257	.7291	.7324	.7357	.7389	.7422	.7454	.7486	.7517	.7549
0.7	.7580	.7611	.7642	.7673	.7704	.7734	.7764	.7794	.7823	.7852
0.8	.7881	.7910	.7939	.7967	.7995	.8023	.8051	.8078	.8106	.8133
0.9	.8159	.8186	.8212	.8238	.8264	.8289	.8315	.8340	.8365	.8389
1.0	.8413	.8438	.8461	.8485	.8508	.8531	.8554	.8577	.8599	.8621
1.1	.8643	.8665	.8686	.8708	.8729	.8749	.8770	.8790	.8810	.8830
1.2	.8849	.8869	.8888	.8907	.8925	.8944	.8962	.8980	.8997	.9015
1.3	.9032	.9049	.9066	.9082	.9099	.9115	.9131	.9147	.9162	.9177
1.4	.9192	.9207	.9222	.9236	.9251	.9265	.9279	.9292	.9306	.9319
1.5	.9332	.9345	.9357	.9370	.9382	.9394	.9406	.9418	.9429	.9441
1.6	.9452	.9463	.9474	.9484	.9495	.9505	.9515	.9525	.9535	.9545
1.7	.9554	.9564	.9573	.9582	.9591	.9599	.9608	.9616	.9625	.9633
1.8	.9641	.9649	.9656	.9664	.9671	.9678	.9686	.9693	.9699	.9706
1.9	.9713	.9719	.9726	.9732	.9738	.9744	.9750	.9756	.9761	.9767
2.0	.9772	.9778	.9783	.9788	.9793	.9798	.9803	.9808	.9812	.9817
2.1	.9821	.9826	.9830	.9834	.9838	.9842	.9846	.9850	.9854	.9857
2.2	.9861	.9864	.9868	.9871	.9875	.9878	.9881	.9884	.9887	.9890
2.3	.9893	.9896	.9898	.9901	.9904	.9906	.9909	.9911	.9913	.9916
2.4	.9918	.9920	.9922	.9925	.9927	.9929	.9931	.9932	.9934	.9936
2.5	.9938	.9940	.9941	.9943	.9945	.9946	.9948	.9949	.9951	.9952
2.6	.9953	.9955	.9956	.9957	.9959	.9960	.9961	.9962	.9963	.9964
2.7	.9965	.9966	.9967	.9968	.9969	.9970	.9971	.9972	.9973	.9974
2.8	.9974	.9975	.9976	.9977	.9977	.9978	.9979	.9979	.9980	.9981
2.9	.9981	.9982	.9982	.9983	.9984	.9984	.9985	.9985	.9986	.9986
3.0	.9987	.9987	.9987	.9988	.9988	.9989	.9989	.9989	.9990	.9990
3.1	.9990	.9991	.9991	.9991	.9992	.9992	.9992	.9992	.9993	.9993
3.2	.9993	.9993	.9994	.9994	.9994	.9994	.9994	.9995	.9995	.9995
3.3	.9995	.9995	.9995	.9996	.9996	.9996	.9996	.9996	.9996	.9997
3.4	.9997	.9997	.9997	.9997	.9997	.9997	.9997	.9997	.9997	.9998
3.5	.9998	.9998	.9998	.9998	.9998	.9998	.9998	.9998	.9998	.9998
3.6	.9998	.9998	.9999	.9999	.9999	.9999	.9999	.9999	.9999	.9999

Table A.2   Critical values of the t-test, i.e. $\tau_{dfs}^{-1}(1 - \alpha)$, with $10 \leq \text{dfs} \leq 40$.

dfs	\multicolumn{8}{c}{Type I error level α}							
	20%	10%	5%	2.5%	1%	0.5%	0.1%	0.05%
10	0.8791	1.3722	1.8125	2.2281	2.6338	3.1693	3.5814	4.5869
11	0.8755	1.3634	1.7959	2.2010	2.5931	3.1058	3.4966	4.4370
12	0.8726	1.3562	1.7823	2.1788	2.5600	3.0545	3.4284	4.3178
13	0.8702	1.3502	1.7709	2.1604	2.5326	3.0123	3.3725	4.2208
14	0.8681	1.3450	1.7613	2.1448	2.5096	2.9768	3.3257	4.1405
15	0.8662	1.3406	1.7531	2.1314	2.4899	2.9467	3.2860	4.0728
16	0.8647	1.3368	1.7459	2.1199	2.4729	2.9208	3.2520	4.0150
17	0.8633	1.3334	1.7396	2.1098	2.4581	2.8982	3.2224	3.9651
18	0.8620	1.3304	1.7341	2.1009	2.4450	2.8784	3.1966	3.9216
19	0.8610	1.3277	1.7291	2.0930	2.4334	2.8609	3.1737	3.8834
20	0.8600	1.3253	1.7247	2.0860	2.4231	2.8453	3.1534	3.8495
21	0.8591	1.3232	1.7207	2.0796	2.4138	2.8314	3.1352	3.8193
22	0.8583	1.3212	1.7171	2.0739	2.4055	2.8188	3.1188	3.7921
23	0.8575	1.3195	1.7139	2.0687	2.3979	2.8073	3.1040	3.7676
24	0.8569	1.3178	1.7109	2.0639	2.3909	2.7969	3.0905	3.7454
25	0.8562	1.3163	1.7081	2.0595	2.3846	2.7874	3.0782	3.7251
26	0.8557	1.3150	1.7056	2.0555	2.3788	2.7787	3.0669	3.7066
27	0.8551	1.3137	1.7033	2.0518	2.3734	2.7707	3.0565	3.6896
28	0.8546	1.3125	1.7011	2.0484	2.3685	2.7633	3.0469	3.6739
29	0.8542	1.3114	1.6991	2.0452	2.3638	2.7564	3.0380	3.6594
30	0.8538	1.3104	1.6973	2.0423	2.3596	2.7500	3.0298	3.6460
31	0.8534	1.3095	1.6955	2.0395	2.3556	2.7440	3.0221	3.6335
32	0.8530	1.3086	1.6939	2.0369	2.3518	2.7385	3.0149	3.6218
33	0.8526	1.3077	1.6924	2.0345	2.3483	2.7333	3.0082	3.6109
34	0.8523	1.3070	1.6909	2.0322	2.3451	2.7284	3.0020	3.6007
35	0.8520	1.3062	1.6896	2.0301	2.3420	2.7238	2.9960	3.5911
36	0.8517	1.3055	1.6883	2.0281	2.3391	2.7195	2.9905	3.5821
37	0.8514	1.3049	1.6871	2.0262	2.3363	2.7154	2.9852	3.5737
38	0.8512	1.3042	1.6860	2.0244	2.3337	2.7116	2.9803	3.5657
39	0.8509	1.3036	1.6849	2.0227	2.3313	2.7079	2.9756	3.5581
40	0.8507	1.3031	1.6839	2.0211	2.3289	2.7045	2.9712	3.5510

Table A.3 Critical values of the t-test, i.e. $\tau_{dfs}^{-1}(1 - \alpha)$, with dfs $\geq$ 40.

dfs	Type I error level α							
	20%	10%	5%	2.5%	1%	0.5%	0.1%	0.05%
40	0.8507	1.3031	1.6839	2.0211	2.3289	2.7045	2.9712	3.5510
42	0.8503	1.3020	1.6820	2.0181	2.3246	2.6981	2.9630	3.5377
44	0.8499	1.3011	1.6802	2.0154	2.3207	2.6923	2.9555	3.5258
46	0.8495	1.3002	1.6787	2.0129	2.3172	2.6870	2.9488	3.5150
48	0.8492	1.2994	1.6772	2.0106	2.3139	2.6822	2.9426	3.5051
50	0.8489	1.2987	1.6759	2.0086	2.3109	2.6778	2.9370	3.4960
55	0.8482	1.2971	1.6730	2.0040	2.3044	2.6682	2.9247	3.4764
60	0.8477	1.2958	1.6706	2.0003	2.2990	2.6603	2.9146	3.4602
65	0.8472	1.2947	1.6686	1.9971	2.2945	2.6536	2.9060	3.4466
70	0.8468	1.2938	1.6669	1.9944	2.2906	2.6479	2.8987	3.4350
75	0.8464	1.2929	1.6654	1.9921	2.2873	2.6430	2.8924	3.4250
80	0.8461	1.2922	1.6641	1.9901	2.2844	2.6387	2.8870	3.4163
85	0.8459	1.2916	1.6630	1.9883	2.2818	2.6349	2.8822	3.4087
90	0.8456	1.2910	1.6620	1.9867	2.2795	2.6316	2.8779	3.4019
95	0.8454	1.2905	1.6611	1.9853	2.2775	2.6286	2.8741	3.3959
100	0.8452	1.2901	1.6602	1.9840	2.2757	2.6259	2.8707	3.3905
110	0.8449	1.2893	1.6588	1.9818	2.2725	2.6213	2.8648	3.3812
120	0.8446	1.2886	1.6577	1.9799	2.2699	2.6174	2.8599	3.3735
130	0.8444	1.2881	1.6567	1.9784	2.2677	2.6142	2.8557	3.3669
140	0.8442	1.2876	1.6558	1.9771	2.2658	2.6114	2.8522	3.3614
150	0.8440	1.2872	1.6551	1.9759	2.2641	2.6090	2.8492	3.3566
175	0.8437	1.2864	1.6536	1.9736	2.2609	2.6042	2.8431	3.3470
200	0.8434	1.2858	1.6525	1.9719	2.2584	2.6006	2.8385	3.3398
250	0.8431	1.2849	1.6510	1.9695	2.2550	2.5956	2.8322	3.3299
300	0.8428	1.2844	1.6499	1.9679	2.2527	2.5923	2.8279	3.3233
400	0.8425	1.2837	1.6487	1.9659	2.2499	2.5882	2.8227	3.3150
500	0.8423	1.2832	1.6479	1.9647	2.2482	2.5857	2.8195	3.3101
750	0.8421	1.2827	1.6469	1.9631	2.2459	2.5824	2.8154	3.3035
1000	0.8420	1.2824	1.6464	1.9623	2.2448	2.5808	2.8133	3.3003
∞	0.8416	1.2816	1.6449	1.9600	2.2414	2.5758	2.8070	3.2905

Table A.4   Critical values of the χ^2-test, i.e. $\chi^2_{dfs}{}^{-1}(1-\alpha)$.

dfs	Type I error level α							
	20%	10%	5%	2.5%	1%	0.5%	0.1%	0.05%
1	1.642	2.706	3.841	5.024	6.635	7.879	10.828	12.116
2	3.219	4.605	5.991	7.378	9.210	10.597	13.816	15.202
3	4.642	6.251	7.815	9.348	11.345	12.838	16.266	17.730
4	5.989	7.779	9.488	11.143	13.277	14.860	18.467	19.997
5	7.289	9.236	11.070	12.833	15.086	16.750	20.515	22.105
6	8.558	10.645	12.592	14.449	16.812	18.548	22.458	24.103
7	9.803	12.017	14.067	16.013	18.475	20.278	24.322	26.018
8	11.030	13.362	15.507	17.535	20.090	21.955	26.124	27.868
9	12.242	14.684	16.919	19.023	21.666	23.589	27.877	29.666
10	13.442	15.987	18.307	20.483	23.209	25.188	29.588	31.420
11	14.631	17.275	19.675	21.920	24.725	26.757	31.264	33.137
12	15.812	18.549	21.026	23.337	26.217	28.300	32.909	34.821
13	16.985	19.812	22.362	24.736	27.688	29.819	34.528	36.478
14	18.151	21.064	23.685	26.119	29.141	31.319	36.123	38.109
15	19.311	22.307	24.996	27.488	30.578	32.801	37.697	39.719
16	20.465	23.542	26.296	28.845	32.000	34.267	39.252	41.308
17	21.615	24.769	27.587	30.191	33.409	35.718	40.790	42.879
18	22.760	25.989	28.869	31.526	34.805	37.156	42.312	44.434
19	23.900	27.204	30.144	32.852	36.191	38.582	43.820	45.973
20	25.038	28.412	31.410	34.170	37.566	39.997	45.315	47.498

Table A.5 Critical values of the Wilcoxon test, i.e. $w_{m,1-\alpha}$, with $m_1 = m_2 = m$, $10 \le m \le 40$.

m	Type I error level α							
	20%	10%	5%	2.5%	1%	0.5%	0.1%	0.05%
10	61	67	72	76	80	83	89	91
11	74	80	86	90	95	99	105	108
12	87	94	101	106	112	116	123	126
13	101	110	117	123	129	134	142	145
14	117	126	134	140	148	153	163	166
15	133	144	152	160	168	173	184	188
16	151	162	172	180	189	195	207	212
17	169	182	192	201	211	218	231	237
18	189	203	214	224	235	242	257	262
19	210	225	237	247	259	267	283	290
20	231	248	261	272	285	294	311	318
21	254	272	286	298	312	322	340	347
22	278	297	312	325	340	350	371	378
23	303	323	339	353	370	380	402	410
24	329	350	368	383	400	411	435	443
25	356	379	397	413	432	444	469	478
26	384	408	428	445	464	477	504	514
27	413	439	460	478	498	512	540	550
28	444	470	492	511	533	548	577	588
29	475	503	526	546	569	585	616	628
30	507	537	561	582	606	623	655	668
31	541	572	597	619	645	662	696	710
32	575	608	635	658	684	702	739	752
33	610	645	673	697	725	744	782	796
34	647	683	712	737	767	786	826	841
35	685	722	753	779	810	830	872	888
36	723	762	794	822	854	875	919	935
37	763	803	837	865	899	921	966	984
38	803	846	880	910	945	968	1016	1034
39	845	889	925	956	992	1016	1066	1085
40	888	934	971	1003	1041	1066	1117	1137

Table A.6 Critical values of the Wilcoxon test, i.e. $w_{m,1-\alpha}$, with $m_1 = m_2 = m$, $41 \leq m \leq 60$.

m	Type I error level α							
	20%	10%	5%	2.5%	1%	0.5%	0.1%	0.05%
41	932	979	1018	1052	1090	1116	1170	1190
42	976	1026	1066	1101	1141	1168	1223	1245
43	1022	1073	1115	1151	1193	1221	1278	1300
44	1069	1122	1165	1203	1246	1275	1334	1357
45	1117	1172	1216	1255	1300	1330	1391	1415
46	1166	1222	1269	1309	1355	1386	1449	1474
47	1216	1274	1322	1363	1411	1443	1509	1534
48	1267	1327	1377	1419	1468	1501	1569	1595
49	1319	1381	1432	1476	1527	1561	1631	1658
50	1373	1436	1489	1534	1586	1622	1694	1722
51	1427	1492	1546	1593	1647	1683	1758	1786
52	1482	1550	1605	1653	1709	1746	1823	1852
53	1538	1608	1665	1714	1771	1810	1889	1919
54	1595	1667	1726	1777	1835	1875	1956	1988
55	1654	1727	1788	1840	1900	1941	2025	2057
56	1713	1789	1851	1904	1966	2008	2094	2127
57	1773	1851	1915	1970	2034	2077	2165	2199
58	1835	1915	1980	2037	2102	2146	2237	2272
59	1897	1979	2046	2104	2171	2217	2310	2346
60	1961	2045	2114	2173	2242	2288	2384	2421

Table A.7   Critical values of the Wilcoxon test, i.e. $w_{m,1-\alpha}$, with sample size rate $k = m_i/m_j = 2, i \neq j, 10 \leq m_j \leq 40$.

m_j	Type I error level α							
	20%	10%	5%	2.5%	1%	0.5%	0.1%	0.05%
10	119	129	137	144	152	157	167	171
11	143	155	164	172	181	187	199	203
12	169	182	193	202	212	219	233	238
13	198	212	224	235	246	254	269	275
14	228	244	258	269	282	291	308	315
15	260	279	293	306	321	330	350	357
16	295	315	331	345	361	372	394	402
17	331	353	371	387	404	416	440	449
18	370	394	414	431	450	463	489	499
19	411	437	458	476	497	511	540	551
20	454	482	505	525	547	562	593	605
21	499	529	554	575	599	616	649	662
22	546	579	605	628	654	671	707	721
23	596	630	658	683	711	729	768	782
24	647	684	714	740	770	790	830	846
25	700	739	771	799	831	852	896	912
26	756	797	831	861	894	917	963	981
27	813	857	893	924	960	984	1033	1052
28	873	919	957	990	1028	1053	1105	1125
29	935	984	1024	1058	1098	1125	1180	1201
30	999	1050	1092	1129	1170	1199	1256	1278
31	1065	1119	1163	1201	1245	1275	1335	1359
32	1133	1189	1236	1276	1322	1353	1417	1441
33	1203	1262	1311	1353	1401	1434	1500	1526
34	1275	1337	1388	1432	1482	1517	1586	1613
35	1349	1414	1467	1513	1566	1602	1675	1703
36	1426	1493	1549	1596	1652	1689	1765	1794
37	1504	1574	1632	1682	1739	1778	1858	1888
38	1585	1658	1718	1770	1830	1870	1953	1985
39	1667	1743	1806	1860	1922	1964	2050	2083
40	1752	1831	1896	1952	2016	2060	2150	2184

APPENDIX B

TABLES OF RP ESTIMATES FOR THE ONE-TAILED z-TEST

Table B.1: Values of the pointwise RP estimates, with $\alpha = 5\%$.

Table B.2: Values of the 90% conservative RP estimates, with $\alpha = 5\%$.

Table B.3: Values of the 95% conservative RP estimates, with $\alpha = 5\%$.

Table B.4: Values of the pointwise RP estimates, with $\alpha = 2.5\%$.

Table B.5: Values of the 90% conservative RP estimates, with $\alpha = 2.5\%$.

Table B.6: Values of the 95% conservative RP estimates, with $\alpha = 2.5\%$.

Table B.7: Values of the pointwise RP estimates, with $\alpha = 1\%$.

Table B.8: Values of the 90% conservative RP estimates, with $\alpha = 1\%$.

Table B.9: Values of the 95% conservative RP estimates, with $\alpha = 1\%$.

Success Probability Estimation with Applications to Clinical Trials, First Edition.
By Daniele De Martini Copyright © 2013 John Wiley & Sons, Inc.

Table B.1 Values (%) of pointwise RP estimates with $\alpha = 5\%$ (i.e. $\hat{RP}_{5\%}$), given the value z of the Gaussian test statistic.

z	0.00	0.01	0.02	0.03	0.04	0.05	0.06	0.07	0.08	0.09
1.6	48.21	48.61	49.01	49.41	49.81	50.21	50.60	51.00	51.40	51.80
1.7	52.20	52.60	53.00	53.39	53.79	54.19	54.58	54.98	55.38	55.77
1.8	56.16	56.56	56.95	57.34	57.74	58.13	58.52	58.91	59.30	59.68
1.9	60.07	60.46	60.84	61.22	61.61	61.99	62.37	62.75	63.12	63.50
2.0	63.88	64.25	64.62	64.99	65.36	65.73	66.10	66.46	66.83	67.19
2.1	67.55	67.91	68.27	68.62	68.98	69.33	69.68	70.03	70.37	70.72
2.2	71.06	71.40	71.74	72.08	72.41	72.75	73.08	73.41	73.73	74.06
2.3	74.38	74.70	75.02	75.34	75.65	75.96	76.27	76.58	76.89	77.19
2.4	77.49	77.79	78.09	78.38	78.67	78.96	79.25	79.54	79.82	80.10
2.5	80.38	80.65	80.93	81.20	81.46	81.73	81.99	82.26	82.51	82.77
2.6	83.02	83.28	83.53	83.77	84.02	84.26	84.50	84.74	84.97	85.20
2.7	85.43	85.66	85.88	86.11	86.33	86.55	86.76	86.97	87.18	87.39
2.8	87.60	87.80	88.00	88.20	88.40	88.59	88.78	88.97	89.16	89.35
2.9	89.53	89.71	89.89	90.06	90.24	90.41	90.58	90.74	90.91	91.07
3.0	91.23	91.39	91.55	91.70	91.85	92.00	92.15	92.29	92.44	92.58
3.1	92.72	92.86	92.99	93.12	93.26	93.39	93.51	93.64	93.76	93.88
3.2	94.00	94.12	94.24	94.35	94.47	94.58	94.69	94.79	94.90	95.00
3.3	95.11	95.21	95.30	95.40	95.50	95.59	95.68	95.77	95.86	95.95
3.4	96.04	96.12	96.21	96.29	96.37	96.45	96.52	96.60	96.68	96.75
3.5	96.82	96.89	96.96	97.03	97.10	97.16	97.23	97.29	97.35	97.41
3.6	97.47	97.53	97.59	97.64	97.70	97.75	97.81	97.86	97.91	97.96
3.7	98.01	98.05	98.10	98.15	98.19	98.24	98.28	98.32	98.36	98.40
3.8	98.44	98.48	98.52	98.56	98.59	98.63	98.66	98.70	98.73	98.76
3.9	98.79	98.82	98.86	98.88	98.91	98.94	98.97	99.00	99.02	99.05
4.0	99.07	99.10	99.12	99.15	99.17	99.19	99.21	99.23	99.26	99.28
4.1	99.30	99.32	99.33	99.35	99.37	99.39	99.41	99.42	99.44	99.45
4.2	99.47	99.48	99.50	99.51	99.53	99.54	99.55	99.57	99.58	99.59
4.3	99.60	99.62	99.63	99.64	99.65	99.66	99.67	99.68	99.69	99.70
4.4	99.71	99.72	99.72	99.73	99.74	99.75	99.76	99.76	99.77	99.78
4.5	99.78	99.79	99.80	99.80	99.81	99.82	99.82	99.83	99.83	99.84
4.6	99.84	99.85	99.85	99.86	99.86	99.87	99.87	99.88	99.88	99.88
4.7	99.89	99.89	99.89	99.90	99.90	99.90	99.91	99.91	99.91	99.92
4.8	99.92	99.92	99.93	99.93	99.93	99.93	99.93	99.94	99.94	99.94
4.9	99.94	99.95	99.95	99.95	99.95	99.95	99.95	99.96	99.96	99.96
5.0	99.96	99.96	99.96	99.96	99.97	99.97	99.97	99.97	99.97	99.97
5.1	99.97	99.97	99.97	99.98	99.98	99.98	99.98	99.98	99.98	99.98
5.2	99.98	99.98	99.98	99.98	99.98	99.98	99.98	99.99	99.99	99.99

Table B.2   Values (%) of 90% conservative RP estimates with $\alpha = 5\%$ (i.e. $\hat{R}P_{5\%}^{90\%}$), given the value z of the Gaussian test statistic.

z	0.00	0.01	0.02	0.03	0.04	0.05	0.06	0.07	0.08	0.09
1.6	9.24	9.40	9.57	9.74	9.92	10.09	10.27	10.45	10.63	10.82
1.7	11.00	11.19	11.38	11.58	11.77	11.97	12.17	12.38	12.58	12.79
1.8	13.00	13.21	13.43	13.65	13.86	14.09	14.31	14.54	14.77	15.00
1.9	15.24	15.47	15.71	15.95	16.20	16.44	16.69	16.94	17.20	17.45
2.0	17.71	17.97	18.24	18.50	18.77	19.04	19.31	19.59	19.87	20.15
2.1	20.43	20.71	21.00	21.29	21.58	21.88	22.17	22.47	22.77	23.07
2.2	23.38	23.69	24.00	24.31	24.62	24.94	25.26	25.58	25.90	26.23
2.3	26.55	26.88	27.21	27.55	27.88	28.22	28.56	28.90	29.24	29.58
2.4	29.93	30.28	30.63	30.98	31.33	31.69	32.05	32.40	32.77	33.13
2.5	33.49	33.86	34.22	34.59	34.96	35.33	35.70	36.08	36.45	36.83
2.6	37.21	37.58	37.96	38.35	38.73	39.11	39.50	39.88	40.27	40.66
2.7	41.04	41.43	41.82	42.21	42.61	43.00	43.39	43.79	44.18	44.58
2.8	44.97	45.37	45.76	46.16	46.56	46.95	47.35	47.75	48.15	48.55
2.9	48.95	49.35	49.74	50.14	50.54	50.94	51.34	51.74	52.14	52.54
3.0	52.93	53.33	53.73	54.13	54.52	54.92	55.31	55.71	56.10	56.50
3.1	56.89	57.28	57.68	58.07	58.46	58.85	59.24	59.62	60.01	60.40
3.2	60.78	61.16	61.55	61.93	62.31	62.69	63.07	63.44	63.82	64.19
3.3	64.56	64.94	65.31	65.67	66.04	66.41	66.77	67.13	67.49	67.85
3.4	68.21	68.57	68.92	69.27	69.62	69.97	70.32	70.66	71.01	71.35
3.5	71.69	72.03	72.36	72.69	73.03	73.36	73.68	74.01	74.33	74.65
3.6	74.97	75.29	75.60	75.92	76.23	76.53	76.84	77.14	77.45	77.74
3.7	78.04	78.34	78.63	78.92	79.21	79.49	79.77	80.06	80.33	80.61
3.8	80.88	81.15	81.42	81.69	81.95	82.22	82.47	82.73	82.99	83.24
3.9	83.49	83.73	83.98	84.22	84.46	84.70	84.93	85.17	85.40	85.62
4.0	85.85	86.07	86.29	86.51	86.73	86.94	87.15	87.36	87.57	87.77
4.1	87.97	88.17	88.37	88.56	88.75	88.94	89.13	89.32	89.50	89.68
4.2	89.86	90.04	90.21	90.38	90.55	90.72	90.88	91.05	91.21	91.37
4.3	91.52	91.68	91.83	91.98	92.13	92.27	92.42	92.56	92.70	92.83
4.4	92.97	93.10	93.24	93.37	93.49	93.62	93.74	93.87	93.99	94.10
4.5	94.22	94.34	94.45	94.56	94.67	94.78	94.88	94.99	95.09	95.19
4.6	95.29	95.39	95.48	95.58	95.67	95.76	95.85	95.94	96.03	96.11
4.7	96.19	96.28	96.36	96.44	96.51	96.59	96.66	96.74	96.81	96.88
4.8	96.95	97.02	97.09	97.15	97.22	97.28	97.34	97.40	97.46	97.52
4.9	97.58	97.63	97.69	97.74	97.80	97.85	97.90	97.95	98.00	98.05
5.0	98.09	98.14	98.19	98.23	98.27	98.31	98.36	98.40	98.44	98.48
5.1	98.51	98.55	98.59	98.62	98.66	98.69	98.72	98.76	98.79	98.82
5.2	98.85	98.88	98.91	98.94	98.97	98.99	99.02	99.05	99.07	99.10

Table B.3   Values (%) of 95% conservative RP estimates with $\alpha = 5\%$ (i.e. $\hat{RP}_{5\%}^{95\%}$), given the value z of the Gaussian test statistic.

z	0.00	0.01	0.02	0.03	0.04	0.05	0.06	0.07	0.08	0.09
1.6	4.55	4.65	4.75	4.85	4.95	5.05	5.16	5.26	5.37	5.48
1.7	5.60	5.71	5.82	5.94	6.06	6.18	6.30	6.43	6.56	6.68
1.8	6.82	6.95	7.08	7.22	7.36	7.50	7.64	7.78	7.93	8.08
1.9	8.23	8.38	8.54	8.70	8.86	9.02	9.18	9.35	9.51	9.69
2.0	9.86	10.03	10.21	10.39	10.57	10.75	10.94	11.13	11.32	11.51
2.1	11.71	11.91	12.11	12.31	12.51	12.72	12.93	13.14	13.36	13.57
2.2	13.79	14.01	14.24	14.46	14.69	14.92	15.16	15.39	15.63	15.87
2.3	16.12	16.36	16.61	16.86	17.11	17.37	17.63	17.89	18.15	18.41
2.4	18.68	18.95	19.22	19.50	19.77	20.05	20.34	20.62	20.91	21.19
2.5	21.48	21.78	22.07	22.37	22.67	22.97	23.28	23.59	23.89	24.21
2.6	24.52	24.83	25.15	25.47	25.79	26.12	26.44	26.77	27.10	27.44
2.7	27.77	28.11	28.44	28.78	29.13	29.47	29.82	30.16	30.51	30.86
2.8	31.22	31.57	31.93	32.29	32.65	33.01	33.37	33.73	34.10	34.47
2.9	34.84	35.21	35.58	35.95	36.33	36.70	37.08	37.46	37.84	38.22
3.0	38.60	38.99	39.37	39.75	40.14	40.53	40.92	41.30	41.69	42.09
3.1	42.48	42.87	43.26	43.66	44.05	44.44	44.84	45.24	45.63	46.03
3.2	46.43	46.82	47.22	47.62	48.02	48.42	48.82	49.21	49.61	50.01
3.3	50.41	50.81	51.21	51.61	52.01	52.40	52.80	53.20	53.60	53.99
3.4	54.39	54.79	55.18	55.58	55.97	56.37	56.76	57.15	57.55	57.94
3.5	58.33	58.72	59.11	59.49	59.88	60.27	60.65	61.04	61.42	61.80
3.6	62.18	62.56	62.94	63.32	63.69	64.07	64.44	64.81	65.18	65.55
3.7	65.92	66.29	66.65	67.01	67.38	67.73	68.09	68.45	68.80	69.16
3.8	69.51	69.86	70.20	70.55	70.89	71.24	71.58	71.91	72.25	72.58
3.9	72.92	73.25	73.57	73.90	74.22	74.55	74.87	75.18	75.50	75.81
4.0	76.12	76.43	76.74	77.04	77.35	77.65	77.94	78.24	78.53	78.82
4.1	79.11	79.40	79.68	79.96	80.24	80.52	80.79	81.06	81.33	81.60
4.2	81.87	82.13	82.39	82.65	82.90	83.15	83.40	83.65	83.90	84.14
4.3	84.38	84.62	84.86	85.09	85.32	85.55	85.78	86.00	86.22	86.44
4.4	86.66	86.87	87.08	87.29	87.50	87.70	87.91	88.11	88.30	88.50
4.5	88.69	88.88	89.07	89.26	89.44	89.62	89.80	89.98	90.15	90.32
4.6	90.50	90.66	90.83	90.99	91.15	91.31	91.47	91.63	91.78	91.93
4.7	92.08	92.22	92.37	92.51	92.65	92.79	92.93	93.06	93.19	93.32
4.8	93.45	93.58	93.70	93.83	93.95	94.07	94.18	94.30	94.41	94.52
4.9	94.63	94.74	94.85	94.95	95.06	95.16	95.26	95.35	95.45	95.55
5.0	95.64	95.73	95.82	95.91	96.00	96.08	96.17	96.25	96.33	96.41
5.1	96.49	96.56	96.64	96.71	96.79	96.86	96.93	97.00	97.06	97.13
5.2	97.20	97.26	97.32	97.38	97.44	97.50	97.56	97.62	97.67	97.73

Table B.4   Values (%) of pointwise RP estimates with $\alpha = 2.5\%$ (i.e. $\hat{RP}_{2.5\%}$), given the value z of the Gaussian test statistic.

z	0.00	0.01	0.02	0.03	0.04	0.05	0.06	0.07	0.08	0.09
1.9	47.61	48.01	48.41	48.80	49.20	49.60	50.00	50.40	50.80	51.20
2.0	51.60	52.00	52.39	52.79	53.19	53.59	53.98	54.38	54.78	55.17
2.1	55.57	55.96	56.36	56.75	57.14	57.54	57.93	58.32	58.71	59.10
2.2	59.48	59.87	60.26	60.64	61.03	61.41	61.79	62.17	62.55	62.93
2.3	63.31	63.68	64.06	64.43	64.80	65.17	65.54	65.91	66.28	66.64
2.4	67.00	67.37	67.73	68.08	68.44	68.79	69.15	69.50	69.85	70.20
2.5	70.54	70.89	71.23	71.57	71.91	72.24	72.58	72.91	73.24	73.57
2.6	73.89	74.22	74.54	74.86	75.18	75.49	75.80	76.12	76.42	76.73
2.7	77.04	77.34	77.64	77.94	78.23	78.52	78.82	79.10	79.39	79.67
2.8	79.96	80.23	80.51	80.79	81.06	81.33	81.59	81.86	82.12	82.38
2.9	82.64	82.90	83.15	83.40	83.65	83.89	84.14	84.38	84.61	84.85
3.0	85.08	85.31	85.54	85.77	85.99	86.22	86.43	86.65	86.87	87.08
3.1	87.29	87.49	87.70	87.90	88.10	88.30	88.49	88.69	88.88	89.07
3.2	89.25	89.44	89.62	89.80	89.97	90.15	90.32	90.49	90.66	90.82
3.3	90.99	91.15	91.31	91.47	91.62	91.77	91.92	92.07	92.22	92.36
3.4	92.51	92.65	92.79	92.92	93.06	93.19	93.32	93.45	93.57	93.70
3.5	93.82	93.94	94.06	94.18	94.30	94.41	94.52	94.63	94.74	94.85
3.6	94.95	95.05	95.15	95.25	95.35	95.45	95.54	95.64	95.73	95.82
3.7	95.91	95.99	96.08	96.16	96.25	96.33	96.41	96.49	96.56	96.64
3.8	96.71	96.78	96.86	96.93	96.99	97.06	97.13	97.19	97.26	97.32
3.9	97.38	97.44	97.50	97.56	97.62	97.67	97.73	97.78	97.83	97.88
4.0	97.93	97.98	98.03	98.08	98.12	98.17	98.21	98.26	98.30	98.34
4.1	98.38	98.42	98.46	98.50	98.54	98.57	98.61	98.64	98.68	98.71
4.2	98.75	98.78	98.81	98.84	98.87	98.90	98.93	98.96	98.98	99.01
4.3	99.04	99.06	99.09	99.11	99.13	99.16	99.18	99.20	99.22	99.25
4.4	99.27	99.29	99.31	99.32	99.34	99.36	99.38	99.40	99.41	99.43
4.5	99.45	99.46	99.48	99.49	99.51	99.52	99.53	99.55	99.56	99.57
4.6	99.59	99.60	99.61	99.62	99.63	99.64	99.65	99.66	99.67	99.68
4.7	99.69	99.70	99.71	99.72	99.73	99.74	99.74	99.75	99.76	99.77
4.8	99.77	99.78	99.79	99.79	99.80	99.81	99.81	99.82	99.83	99.83
4.9	99.84	99.84	99.85	99.85	99.86	99.86	99.87	99.87	99.87	99.88
5.0	99.88	99.89	99.89	99.89	99.90	99.90	99.90	99.91	99.91	99.91
5.1	99.92	99.92	99.92	99.92	99.93	99.93	99.93	99.93	99.94	99.94
5.2	99.94	99.94	99.94	99.95	99.95	99.95	99.95	99.95	99.95	99.96
5.3	99.96	99.96	99.96	99.96	99.96	99.97	99.97	99.97	99.97	99.97
5.4	99.97	99.97	99.97	99.97	99.97	99.98	99.98	99.98	99.98	99.98
5.5	99.98	99.98	99.98	99.98	99.98	99.98	99.98	99.98	99.99	99.99

Table B.5   Values (%) of 90% conservative RP estimates with $\alpha = 2.5\%$ (i.e. $\hat{RP}^{90\%}_{2.5\%}$), given the value z of the Gaussian test statistic.

z	0.00	0.01	0.02	0.03	0.04	0.05	0.06	0.07	0.08	0.09
1.9	8.99	9.15	9.32	9.48	9.65	9.83	10.00	10.18	10.36	10.54
2.0	10.72	10.91	11.09	11.28	11.48	11.67	11.87	12.07	12.27	12.48
2.1	12.68	12.89	13.10	13.32	13.53	13.75	13.97	14.20	14.42	14.65
2.2	14.88	15.11	15.35	15.59	15.83	16.07	16.32	16.56	16.81	17.07
2.3	17.32	17.58	17.84	18.10	18.37	18.63	18.90	19.17	19.45	19.72
2.4	20.00	20.28	20.57	20.85	21.14	21.43	21.72	22.02	22.32	22.62
2.5	22.92	23.22	23.53	23.84	24.15	24.46	24.78	25.09	25.41	25.74
2.6	26.06	26.39	26.71	27.04	27.37	27.71	28.04	28.38	28.72	29.06
2.7	29.41	29.75	30.10	30.45	30.80	31.15	31.51	31.86	32.22	32.58
2.8	32.94	33.30	33.67	34.03	34.40	34.77	35.14	35.51	35.89	36.26
2.9	36.64	37.01	37.39	37.77	38.15	38.53	38.92	39.30	39.68	40.07
3.0	40.46	40.85	41.23	41.62	42.01	42.41	42.80	43.19	43.58	43.98
3.1	44.37	44.77	45.16	45.56	45.96	46.35	46.75	47.15	47.55	47.95
3.2	48.34	48.74	49.14	49.54	49.94	50.34	50.74	51.14	51.53	51.93
3.3	52.33	52.73	53.13	53.53	53.92	54.32	54.72	55.11	55.51	55.90
3.4	56.30	56.69	57.08	57.48	57.87	58.26	58.65	59.04	59.42	59.81
3.5	60.20	60.58	60.97	61.35	61.73	62.11	62.49	62.87	63.25	63.63
3.6	64.00	64.37	64.75	65.12	65.49	65.85	66.22	66.59	66.95	67.31
3.7	67.67	68.03	68.38	68.74	69.09	69.44	69.79	70.14	70.49	70.83
3.8	71.17	71.51	71.85	72.19	72.52	72.86	73.19	73.52	73.84	74.17
3.9	74.49	74.81	75.13	75.44	75.76	76.07	76.38	76.68	76.99	77.29
4.0	77.59	77.89	78.19	78.48	78.77	79.06	79.35	79.63	79.91	80.19
4.1	80.47	80.74	81.02	81.29	81.55	81.82	82.08	82.34	82.60	82.86
4.2	83.11	83.36	83.61	83.85	84.10	84.34	84.58	84.81	85.05	85.28
4.3	85.51	85.73	85.96	86.18	86.40	86.62	86.83	87.04	87.25	87.46
4.4	87.67	87.87	88.07	88.27	88.46	88.66	88.85	89.04	89.22	89.41
4.5	89.59	89.77	89.95	90.12	90.29	90.46	90.63	90.80	90.96	91.12
4.6	91.28	91.44	91.60	91.75	91.90	92.05	92.20	92.34	92.49	92.63
4.7	92.76	92.90	93.04	93.17	93.30	93.43	93.56	93.68	93.80	93.92
4.8	94.04	94.16	94.28	94.39	94.50	94.61	94.72	94.83	94.93	95.04
4.9	95.14	95.24	95.34	95.43	95.53	95.62	95.71	95.80	95.89	95.98
5.0	96.07	96.15	96.23	96.32	96.39	96.47	96.55	96.63	96.70	96.77
5.1	96.84	96.92	96.98	97.05	97.12	97.18	97.25	97.31	97.37	97.43
5.2	97.49	97.55	97.61	97.66	97.72	97.77	97.82	97.87	97.92	97.97
5.3	98.02	98.07	98.12	98.16	98.21	98.25	98.29	98.34	98.38	98.42
5.4	98.46	98.49	98.53	98.57	98.60	98.64	98.67	98.71	98.74	98.77
5.5	98.80	98.84	98.87	98.89	98.92	98.95	98.98	99.01	99.03	99.06

Table B.6 Values (%) of 95% conservative RP estimates with $\alpha = 2.5\%$ (i.e. $\hat{RP}^{95\%}_{2.5\%}$), given the value z of the Gaussian test statistic.

z	0.00	0.01	0.02	0.03	0.04	0.05	0.06	0.07	0.08	0.09
1.9	4.41	4.51	4.60	4.70	4.80	4.90	5.00	5.10	5.21	5.32
2.0	5.43	5.54	5.65	5.76	5.88	6.00	6.12	6.24	6.37	6.49
2.1	6.62	6.75	6.88	7.01	7.15	7.29	7.43	7.57	7.71	7.86
2.2	8.00	8.15	8.31	8.46	8.62	8.77	8.93	9.10	9.26	9.43
2.3	9.60	9.77	9.94	10.12	10.30	10.48	10.66	10.84	11.03	11.22
2.4	11.41	11.61	11.80	12.00	12.20	12.41	12.61	12.82	13.03	13.25
2.5	13.46	13.68	13.90	14.12	14.35	14.58	14.81	15.04	15.27	15.51
2.6	15.75	15.99	16.24	16.48	16.73	16.98	17.24	17.49	17.75	18.01
2.7	18.28	18.54	18.81	19.08	19.36	19.63	19.91	20.19	20.47	20.76
2.8	21.05	21.34	21.63	21.92	22.22	22.52	22.82	23.12	23.43	23.74
2.9	24.05	24.36	24.67	24.99	25.31	25.63	25.95	26.28	26.60	26.93
3.0	27.27	27.60	27.93	28.27	28.61	28.95	29.29	29.64	29.99	30.33
3.1	30.68	31.04	31.39	31.75	32.10	32.46	32.82	33.18	33.55	33.91
3.2	34.28	34.65	35.02	35.39	35.76	36.14	36.51	36.89	37.27	37.65
3.3	38.03	38.41	38.79	39.17	39.56	39.94	40.33	40.72	41.11	41.50
3.4	41.89	42.28	42.67	43.06	43.45	43.85	44.24	44.64	45.03	45.43
3.5	45.83	46.22	46.62	47.02	47.42	47.81	48.21	48.61	49.01	49.41
3.6	49.81	50.21	50.61	51.00	51.40	51.80	52.20	52.60	53.00	53.39
3.7	53.79	54.19	54.58	54.98	55.38	55.77	56.17	56.56	56.95	57.35
3.8	57.74	58.13	58.52	58.91	59.30	59.68	60.07	60.46	60.84	61.22
3.9	61.61	61.99	62.37	62.75	63.13	63.50	63.88	64.25	64.62	64.99
4.0	65.36	65.73	66.10	66.46	66.83	67.19	67.55	67.91	68.27	68.62
4.1	68.98	69.33	69.68	70.03	70.37	70.72	71.06	71.40	71.74	72.08
4.2	72.41	72.75	73.08	73.41	73.73	74.06	74.38	74.70	75.02	75.34
4.3	75.65	75.97	76.28	76.58	76.89	77.19	77.49	77.79	78.09	78.38
4.4	78.67	78.96	79.25	79.54	79.82	80.10	80.38	80.65	80.93	81.20
4.5	81.47	81.73	82.00	82.26	82.52	82.77	83.03	83.28	83.53	83.77
4.6	84.02	84.26	84.50	84.74	84.97	85.20	85.43	85.66	85.89	86.11
4.7	86.33	86.55	86.76	86.97	87.19	87.39	87.60	87.80	88.00	88.20
4.8	88.40	88.59	88.79	88.97	89.16	89.35	89.53	89.71	89.89	90.06
4.9	90.24	90.41	90.58	90.74	90.91	91.07	91.23	91.39	91.55	91.70
5.0	91.85	92.00	92.15	92.29	92.44	92.58	92.72	92.86	92.99	93.13
5.1	93.26	93.39	93.51	93.64	93.76	93.88	94.00	94.12	94.24	94.35
5.2	94.47	94.58	94.69	94.79	94.90	95.00	95.11	95.21	95.31	95.40
5.3	95.50	95.59	95.68	95.78	95.86	95.95	96.04	96.12	96.21	96.29
5.4	96.37	96.45	96.53	96.60	96.68	96.75	96.82	96.89	96.96	97.03
5.5	97.10	97.16	97.23	97.29	97.35	97.41	97.47	97.53	97.59	97.64

Table B.7   Values (%) of pointwise RP estimates with $\alpha = 1\%$ (i.e. $\hat{RP}_{1\%}$), given the value z of the Gaussian test statistic.

z	0.00	0.01	0.02	0.03	0.04	0.05	0.06	0.07	0.08	0.09
2.3	48.95	49.35	49.75	50.15	50.54	50.94	51.34	51.74	52.14	52.54
2.4	52.94	53.33	53.73	54.13	54.52	54.92	55.32	55.71	56.11	56.50
2.5	56.89	57.29	57.68	58.07	58.46	58.85	59.24	59.62	60.01	60.40
2.6	60.78	61.17	61.55	61.93	62.31	62.69	63.07	63.44	63.82	64.19
2.7	64.57	64.94	65.31	65.68	66.04	66.41	66.77	67.14	67.50	67.86
2.8	68.21	68.57	68.92	69.27	69.63	69.97	70.32	70.67	71.01	71.35
2.9	71.69	72.03	72.36	72.70	73.03	73.36	73.68	74.01	74.33	74.65
3.0	74.97	75.29	75.60	75.92	76.23	76.54	76.84	77.15	77.45	77.75
3.1	78.04	78.34	78.63	78.92	79.21	79.49	79.78	80.06	80.34	80.61
3.2	80.88	81.16	81.42	81.69	81.96	82.22	82.48	82.73	82.99	83.24
3.3	83.49	83.74	83.98	84.22	84.46	84.70	84.94	85.17	85.40	85.63
3.4	85.85	86.07	86.29	86.51	86.73	86.94	87.15	87.36	87.57	87.77
3.5	87.97	88.17	88.37	88.56	88.76	88.95	89.13	89.32	89.50	89.68
3.6	89.86	90.04	90.21	90.38	90.55	90.72	90.88	91.05	91.21	91.37
3.7	91.52	91.68	91.83	91.98	92.13	92.27	92.42	92.56	92.70	92.84
3.8	92.97	93.10	93.24	93.37	93.49	93.62	93.74	93.87	93.99	94.11
3.9	94.22	94.34	94.45	94.56	94.67	94.78	94.88	94.99	95.09	95.19
4.0	95.29	95.39	95.48	95.58	95.67	95.76	95.85	95.94	96.03	96.11
4.1	96.19	96.28	96.36	96.44	96.51	96.59	96.66	96.74	96.81	96.88
4.2	96.95	97.02	97.09	97.15	97.22	97.28	97.34	97.40	97.46	97.52
4.3	97.58	97.64	97.69	97.74	97.80	97.85	97.90	97.95	98.00	98.05
4.4	98.09	98.14	98.19	98.23	98.27	98.32	98.36	98.40	98.44	98.48
4.5	98.51	98.55	98.59	98.62	98.66	98.69	98.72	98.76	98.79	98.82
4.6	98.85	98.88	98.91	98.94	98.97	98.99	99.02	99.05	99.07	99.10
4.7	99.12	99.14	99.17	99.19	99.21	99.23	99.25	99.27	99.29	99.31
4.8	99.33	99.35	99.37	99.39	99.40	99.42	99.44	99.45	99.47	99.48
4.9	99.50	99.51	99.53	99.54	99.55	99.57	99.58	99.59	99.60	99.61
5.0	99.62	99.64	99.65	99.66	99.67	99.68	99.69	99.70	99.71	99.71
5.1	99.72	99.73	99.74	99.75	99.76	99.76	99.77	99.78	99.78	99.79
5.2	99.80	99.80	99.81	99.82	99.82	99.83	99.83	99.84	99.84	99.85
5.3	99.85	99.86	99.86	99.87	99.87	99.88	99.88	99.88	99.89	99.89
5.4	99.89	99.90	99.90	99.90	99.91	99.91	99.91	99.92	99.92	99.92
5.5	99.92	99.93	99.93	99.93	99.93	99.94	99.94	99.94	99.94	99.95
5.6	99.95	99.95	99.95	99.95	99.95	99.96	99.96	99.96	99.96	99.96
5.7	99.96	99.96	99.97	99.97	99.97	99.97	99.97	99.97	99.97	99.97
5.8	99.97	99.98	99.98	99.98	99.98	99.98	99.98	99.98	99.98	99.98
5.9	99.98	99.98	99.98	99.98	99.98	99.99	99.99	99.99	99.99	99.99

Table B.8 Values (%) of 90% conservative RP estimates with $\alpha = 1\%$ (i.e. $\hat{RP}_{1\%}^{90\%}$), given the value z of the Gaussian test statistic.

z	0.00	0.01	0.02	0.03	0.04	0.05	0.06	0.07	0.08	0.09
2.3	9.55	9.72	9.89	10.06	10.24	10.42	10.60	10.79	10.97	11.16
2.4	11.35	11.55	11.74	11.94	12.14	12.35	12.55	12.76	12.97	13.18
2.5	13.40	13.61	13.83	14.05	14.28	14.51	14.73	14.97	15.20	15.44
2.6	15.68	15.92	16.16	16.41	16.65	16.91	17.16	17.41	17.67	17.93
2.7	18.20	18.46	18.73	19.00	19.27	19.55	19.82	20.10	20.39	20.67
2.8	20.96	21.25	21.54	21.83	22.13	22.43	22.73	23.03	23.33	23.64
2.9	23.95	24.26	24.58	24.89	25.21	25.53	25.85	26.18	26.50	26.83
3.0	27.16	27.50	27.83	28.17	28.51	28.85	29.19	29.53	29.88	30.23
3.1	30.58	30.93	31.28	31.64	31.99	32.35	32.71	33.07	33.44	33.80
3.2	34.17	34.54	34.90	35.28	35.65	36.02	36.40	36.77	37.15	37.53
3.3	37.91	38.29	38.67	39.05	39.44	39.82	40.21	40.60	40.99	41.38
3.4	41.77	42.16	42.55	42.94	43.33	43.73	44.12	44.52	44.91	45.31
3.5	45.70	46.10	46.50	46.90	47.29	47.69	48.09	48.49	48.89	49.29
3.6	49.68	50.08	50.48	50.88	51.28	51.68	52.08	52.48	52.87	53.27
3.7	53.67	54.07	54.46	54.86	55.25	55.65	56.04	56.44	56.83	57.22
3.8	57.62	58.01	58.40	58.79	59.18	59.56	59.95	60.34	60.72	61.11
3.9	61.49	61.87	62.25	62.63	63.01	63.39	63.76	64.14	64.51	64.88
4.0	65.25	65.62	65.99	66.35	66.72	67.08	67.44	67.80	68.16	68.51
4.1	68.87	69.22	69.57	69.92	70.27	70.61	70.96	71.30	71.64	71.98
4.2	72.31	72.64	72.98	73.31	73.63	73.96	74.28	74.60	74.92	75.24
4.3	75.56	75.87	76.18	76.49	76.79	77.10	77.40	77.70	78.00	78.29
4.4	78.58	78.88	79.16	79.45	79.73	80.01	80.29	80.57	80.84	81.11
4.5	81.38	81.65	81.91	82.18	82.44	82.69	82.95	83.20	83.45	83.70
4.6	83.94	84.19	84.43	84.66	84.90	85.13	85.36	85.59	85.82	86.04
4.7	86.26	86.48	86.70	86.91	87.12	87.33	87.54	87.74	87.94	88.14
4.8	88.34	88.53	88.73	88.92	89.10	89.29	89.47	89.65	89.83	90.01
4.9	90.18	90.36	90.53	90.69	90.86	91.02	91.18	91.34	91.50	91.65
5.0	91.81	91.96	92.10	92.25	92.39	92.54	92.68	92.81	92.95	93.08
5.1	93.22	93.35	93.47	93.60	93.73	93.85	93.97	94.09	94.20	94.32
5.2	94.43	94.54	94.65	94.76	94.87	94.97	95.07	95.18	95.27	95.37
5.3	95.47	95.56	95.66	95.75	95.84	95.93	96.01	96.10	96.18	96.26
5.4	96.34	96.42	96.50	96.58	96.65	96.73	96.80	96.87	96.94	97.01
5.5	97.08	97.14	97.21	97.27	97.33	97.39	97.45	97.51	97.57	97.63
5.6	97.68	97.74	97.79	97.84	97.89	97.94	97.99	98.04	98.09	98.13
5.7	98.18	98.22	98.27	98.31	98.35	98.39	98.43	98.47	98.51	98.54
5.8	98.58	98.62	98.65	98.69	98.72	98.75	98.78	98.82	98.85	98.88
5.9	98.91	98.93	98.96	98.99	99.02	99.04	99.07	99.09	99.12	99.14

Table B.9 Values (%) of 95% conservative RP estimates with $\alpha = 1\%$ (i.e. $\widehat{RP}_{1\%}^{95\%}$), given the value z of the Gaussian test statistic.

z	0.00	0.01	0.02	0.03	0.04	0.05	0.06	0.07	0.08	0.09
2.3	4.73	4.83	4.93	5.04	5.14	5.25	5.36	5.47	5.58	5.69
2.4	5.81	5.92	6.04	6.16	6.29	6.41	6.54	6.67	6.80	6.93
2.5	7.06	7.20	7.34	7.48	7.62	7.76	7.91	8.06	8.21	8.36
2.6	8.52	8.67	8.83	8.99	9.16	9.32	9.49	9.66	9.83	10.01
2.7	10.18	10.36	10.54	10.73	10.91	11.10	11.29	11.48	11.68	11.88
2.8	12.08	12.28	12.48	12.69	12.90	13.11	13.32	13.54	13.76	13.98
2.9	14.20	14.43	14.66	14.89	15.12	15.36	15.60	15.84	16.08	16.32
3.0	16.57	16.82	17.08	17.33	17.59	17.85	18.11	18.37	18.64	18.91
3.1	19.18	19.46	19.73	20.01	20.29	20.58	20.86	21.15	21.44	21.73
3.2	22.03	22.33	22.63	22.93	23.23	23.54	23.85	24.16	24.47	24.79
3.3	25.10	25.42	25.75	26.07	26.40	26.72	27.05	27.39	27.72	28.06
3.4	28.39	28.73	29.07	29.42	29.76	30.11	30.46	30.81	31.16	31.52
3.5	31.87	32.23	32.59	32.95	33.32	33.68	34.05	34.41	34.78	35.15
3.6	35.52	35.90	36.27	36.65	37.02	37.40	37.78	38.16	38.54	38.93
3.7	39.31	39.70	40.08	40.47	40.86	41.25	41.64	42.03	42.42	42.81
3.8	43.20	43.60	43.99	44.39	44.78	45.18	45.57	45.97	46.37	46.76
3.9	47.16	47.56	47.96	48.36	48.76	49.15	49.55	49.95	50.35	50.75
4.0	51.15	51.55	51.95	52.34	52.74	53.14	53.54	53.94	54.33	54.73
4.1	55.12	55.52	55.91	56.31	56.70	57.10	57.49	57.88	58.27	58.66
4.2	59.05	59.44	59.82	60.21	60.60	60.98	61.36	61.75	62.13	62.51
4.3	62.88	63.26	63.64	64.01	64.39	64.76	65.13	65.50	65.87	66.23
4.4	66.60	66.96	67.32	67.68	68.04	68.40	68.75	69.10	69.46	69.80
4.5	70.15	70.50	70.84	71.19	71.53	71.86	72.20	72.53	72.87	73.20
4.6	73.53	73.85	74.18	74.50	74.82	75.14	75.45	75.77	76.08	76.39
4.7	76.69	77.00	77.30	77.60	77.90	78.20	78.49	78.78	79.07	79.35
4.8	79.64	79.92	80.20	80.48	80.75	81.02	81.29	81.56	81.83	82.09
4.9	82.35	82.61	82.86	83.12	83.37	83.62	83.86	84.11	84.35	84.59
5.0	84.82	85.06	85.29	85.52	85.74	85.97	86.19	86.41	86.62	86.84
5.1	87.05	87.26	87.47	87.67	87.88	88.08	88.27	88.47	88.66	88.85
5.2	89.04	89.23	89.41	89.59	89.77	89.95	90.13	90.30	90.47	90.64
5.3	90.80	90.97	91.13	91.29	91.45	91.60	91.76	91.91	92.06	92.20
5.4	92.35	92.49	92.63	92.77	92.91	93.04	93.17	93.30	93.43	93.56
5.5	93.68	93.81	93.93	94.05	94.17	94.28	94.39	94.51	94.62	94.73
5.6	94.83	94.94	95.04	95.14	95.24	95.34	95.44	95.53	95.63	95.72
5.7	95.81	95.90	95.98	96.07	96.15	96.24	96.32	96.40	96.48	96.55
5.8	96.63	96.70	96.78	96.85	96.92	96.99	97.05	97.12	97.19	97.25
5.9	97.31	97.37	97.43	97.49	97.55	97.61	97.66	97.72	97.77	97.82

REFERENCES

1. A. Agresti. A survey of exact inference for Contingency Tables. *Statistical Science*, Vol. 7(1): 131-177, 1992.

2. A. Agresti. *Categorical Data Analysis*. Wiley, Hoboken, 2nd ed. 2002.

3. A. Agresti, C.R. Mehta, and N.R. Patel. Exact Inference for Contingency Tables with Ordered Categories. *Journal of the American Statistical Association*, Vol. 85(410): 453-458, 1990.

4. M.A. Arcones and E. Giné. On the bootstrap of U and V statistics. *Annals of Statistics*, Vol. 20(2): 655-674, 1992.

5. R.L. Berger. More powerful tests from confidence interval p values. *American Statistician*, Vol. 50(4): 314-318, 1996.

6. A. Berger, J.T. Wittes, and R.Z. Gold. On the Power of the Cochran-Mantel-Haenszel Test and of Other Approximately Optimal Tests for Partial Association. *Technical Report B-03, Columbia University School of Public Health, Division of Biostatistics*, 1979.

7. R.C. Blair and J.J. Higgins. A Comparison of the Power of Wilcoxon's Rank-Sum Statistic to that of Student's *t*-Statistic Under Various Nonnormal Distributions. *Journal of Educational and Behavioral Statistics*, Vol. 5: 309-335, 1980.

8. G.E. Box, H.G. Hunter, and J.S. Hunter. *Statistics for experimenters: an introduction to design, data analysis, and model building*. Wiley, Hoboken, 2nd ed. 2005.

9. H. Breslow. A generalized Kruskal-Wallis test for comparing K samples subject to unequal patterns of censorship. *Biometrika*, Vol. 57(3): 579-594, 1970.

10. E. Brittain and J.J. Schlesselman. Optimal Allocation for the Comparison of Proportions. *Biometrics*, Vol. 38(4): 1003-1009, 1982.

11. C. Chuang-Stein. Sample Size and the Probability of a Successful Trial. *Pharmaceutical Statistics*, Vol. 5(4): 305-309, 2006

12. D. Collett. *Modelling Survival Data in Medical Research*. CRC Press, Boca Raton, 2003.

13. W.J. Conover. *Practical Nonparametric Statistics*. John Wiley & Sons, New York, 3rd ed. 1999.

14. P.F. Darken and S.Y. Ho. A note on sample size savings with the use of a single well-controlled clinical trial to support the efficacy of a new drug. *Pharmaceutical Statistics*, Vol. 3(1): 61-63, 2004

15. L. De Capitani and D. De Martini. On stochastic orderings of the Wilcoxon Rank Sum test statistic - with applications to reproducibility probability estimation testing. *Statistics and Probability Letters*, Vol. 81(8): 937-946, 2011.

16. L. De Capitani and D. De Martini. Reproducibility probability estimation and testing for the Wilcoxon rank-sum test. WP, 2012.

17. D. De Martini. Smoothed bootstrap consistency through the convergence in mallows metric of smooth estimates. *Journal of Nonparametric Statistics*, Vol. 12(6): 819-835, 2000.

18. D. De Martini. Reproducibility probability estimation for testing statistical hypotheses. *Statistics and Probability Letters*, Vol. 78(9): 1056-1061, 2008.

19. D. De Martini. Conservative Sample Size Estimation in Nonparametrics. *Journal of Biopharmaceutical Statistics*, Vol. 21(1): 24-41, 2011a.

20. D. De Martini. Adapting by calibration the sample size of a phase III trial on the basis of phase II data. *Pharmaceutical Statistics*, Vol. 10(2): 89-95, 2011b.

21. D. De Martini. Robustness and corrections for sample size adaptation strategies based on effect size estimation. *Communications in Statistics - Simulation and Computation*, Vol. 40(9): 1263-1277, 2011c.

22. D. De Martini. Stability Criteria for the Outcomes of Statistical Tests to Assess Drug Effectiveness with a Single Study. *Pharmaceutical Statistics*, Vol. 11(4): 273-279, 2012.

23. K.R. Eberhardt and M.A. Fligner. Comparison of Two Tests for Equality of Two Proportions. *American Statistician*, Vol. 31(4): 151-155, 1977.

24. B. Efron and R.J. Tibshirani. *An introduction to the Bootstrap*. Chapman & Hall, New York, 1993.

25. EMEA, The European Agency for Evaluation of Medicinal Products. Note for Guidance on Statistical Principles for Clinical Trials. International Conference on Harmonization - Topic E 9. 1998.

26. EMEA, The European Agency for Evaluation of Medicinal Products. Committee for Proprietary Medicinal Products (CPMP). Points to Consider on Application with 1. Meta-Analyses; 2. One Pivotal Study. 2001.

27. M.P. Fay, M.E. Halloran, and D.A. Follmann. Accounting for Variability in Sample Size Estimation with Applications to Nonhaderence and Estimation of Variance and Effect Size. *Biometrics* Vol. 63(2): 465-474, 2007.

28. FDA, Food and Drug Administration, Modernization Act, Sec. 115. 1997.

29. FDA, Food and Drug Administration (CDER-CBER), and U.S. Department of Health and Human Services. Guideline for Industry - Providing Clinical Evidence of Effectiveness for Human Drugs and Biological Products. 1998.

30. R.A. Fisher. On the Interpretation of χ^2 from Contingency Tables, and the Calculation of P. *Journal of the Royal Statistical Society*, Vol. 85(1): 87-94, 1922

31. C. Forbes, M. Evans, N. Hastings, and B. Peacock. *Statistical Distributions*. John Wiley & Sons, Hoboken, 4th ed. 2011.

32. M. Gail. The Determination of Sample Sizes for Trials Involving Several Independent 2 x 2 Tables. *Journal of Chronic Diseases*, Vol. 26: 669-673, 1973.

33. J.D. Gibbons and S. Chakraborti. *Nonparametric Statistical Inference*, Dekker, New York, 4th ed. 2003.

34. S.N. Goodman. A comment on replication, p-values and evidence. *Statistics in Medicine*, Vol. 11(7): 875-879, 1992.

35. Guidance for Industry: ICH, International Conference on Harmonization. (1998). Guidance on Statistical Principles for Clinical Trials - E9. Federal Register, Vol. 63, No.179, 49583-49598.

36. P. Hall and M.A. Martin. On bootstrap Resampling and Iteration. *Biometrika*, Vol. 75(4): 661-671, 1988.

37. H.L. Harter. Error Rates and Sample Sizes for Range Tests in Multiple Comparisons. *Biometrics*, Vol. 13: 511-536, 1957.

38. C. Hirotsu. Cumulative chi-squared Statistic as a Tool for Testing Goodness of Fit. *Biometrika*, Vol. 73(1): 165-173, 1986.

39. W. Hoeffding. The Large Sample Power of Test Based on Permutations of Observations. *Annals of Mathematical Statistics*, Vol. 23: 169-192, 1952.

40. H.M.J. Hung and R.T. O'Neill. Utilities of the P-value Distribution Associated with Effect Size in Clinical Trials. *Biometrical Journal*, Vol. 45(6): 659-669, 2003.

41. H.M.J. Hung, S.J. Wang, and R.T. O'Neill. Methodological issues with adaptation of clinical trial design. *Pharmaceutical Statistics*, Vol. 5(2): 99-107, 2006.

42. R.I. Jennrich. Some exact tests for comparing survival curves in the presence of unequal right censoring. *Biometrika*, Vol. 71(1): 57-64, 1984.

43. J.M. Lachin. Sample Size Determinations for r x c Comparative Trials. *Biometrics*, Vol. 33(2): 315-324, 1977.

44. E.L. Lehmann. *Nonparametrics: statistical methods based on ranks*. Holden Day, San Francisco, 1975.

45. E.L. Lehmann and J.P. Romano. *Testing statistical hypotheses*. Springer, New York, 3rd ed. 2005.

46. A. Lucadamo, N. Accoto, and D. De Martini. Power Estimation for Multiple Co-Primary Endpoints: a comparison among conservative solutions. *Italian Journal of Public Health*, Vol. 4, 2012.

47. M.A. Martin. On the double bootstrap. *Technical Report No. 347, Department of Statistics, Stanford University*, 1990.

48. K. McCartney and R. Rosenthal. Effect Size, Practical Importance, and Social Policy for Children. *Child Development*, Vol. 71(1): 173-180, 2000.

49. P. McCullagh and J.A. Nelder. *Generalized Linear Models*. Chapman and Hall, London, 1989.

50. A. Munoz and B. Rosner. Power and Sample Size for a Collection of 2 x 2 Tables. *Biometrics*, Vol. 40(4): 995-1004, 1984.

51. R.G. Newcombe. Confidence intervals for an effect size measure based on the Mann-Whitney statistic. Part 1: General issues and tail-area-based methods. *Statistics in Medicine* Vol. 25(4): 543-557, 2006a.

52. R.G. Newcombe. Confidence intervals for an effect size measure based on the Mann-Whitney statistic. Part 2: Asymptotic methods and evaluation. *Statistics in Medicine* Vol. 25(4): 559-573, 2006b.

53. G.E. Noether. Sample size determination for some common nonparametric tests. *Journal of the American Statistical Association* Vol. 82(398): 645-647, 1987.

54. K.J. Ottenbacher. The Power of Replications and Replications of Power. *The American Statistician* Vol. 50(3): 271-275, 1996.

55. M. Pagano and D. Tritchler. Algorithms for the analysis of several 2 x 2 contingency tables. *SIAM Journal of Scientific and Statistical Computing*, Vol. 4(2): 302-309, 1983a.

56. M. Pagano and D. Tritchler. On obtaining permutation distributions in polynomial time. *Journal of the American Statistical Association*, Vol. 78(382): 435-440, 1983b.

57. B. Rosner. *Fundamentals of Biostatistics*. Duxbury Press, Boston, 6th ed. 2005.

58. S.R. Searle. *Linear Models*. John Wiley & Sons, New York, 1971.

59. H. Scheffé. Practical Solutions of the Behrens-Fisher Problem. *Journal of the American Statistical Association*, Vol. 65(332): 1501-1508, 1970.

60. H. Scheffé. *The Analysis of Variance*. Wiley Classic Library Edition, New York, 1999.

61. R.J. Serfling. *Approximation Theorems of Mathematical Statistics*. Wiley, New York, 1980.

62. J. Shao and S.C. Chow. Reproducibility probability in clinical trials. *Statistics in Medicine* Vol. 21(12): 1727-1742, 2002.

63. Z. Shun, E. Chi, S. Durrleman, and L. Fisher. Statistical consideration on the strategy for demonstrating clinical evidence of effectiveness - one larger vs two smaller pivotal studies. *Statistics in Medicine*, Vol. 24(11): 1619-1637, 2005.

64. B.W. Silverman. *Density Estimation for Statistics and Data Analysis*. Chapman and Hall, New York, 1986.

65. H. Wang, B. Chen, and S.C. Chow. Sample size determination based on rank tests in clinical trials. *Journal of Biopharmaceutical Statistics*, Vol. 13(4): 735-751, 2003.

66. S.J. Wang, H.M.J. Hung, and R.T. O'Neill. Adapting the sample size planning of a phase III trial based on phase II data. *Pharmaceutical Statistics*, Vol. 5(2): 85-97, 2006.

67. B.L. Welch. The Generalization of 'Student's' Problem When Several Different Population Variances Are Involved. *Biometrika*, Vol. 34(1/2): 28-35, 1947.

68. B.L. Welch. Further Note on Mrs. Aspin's Tables and on Certain Approximations to the Tabled Function. *Biometrika*, Vol. 36: 293-296, 1949.

69. J.T. Wittes and S. Wallenstein. The Power of the Mantel-Haenszel Test. *Journal of the American Statistical Association*, Vol. 82(400): 1104-1109, 1987.

70. D. Zhang and H. Quan. Power and sample size calculation for log-rank test with a time lag in treatment effect. *Statistics in Medicine* Vol. 28(5): 864-879, 2009.

TOPIC INDEX

A

adaptation, 58
alternative hypothesis, 10
    of clinical equivalence, 23, 24
    of clinical non-inferiority, 23
    of clinical superiority, 23
    of inequality, 20
    of superiority, 10
asterisk scale, 34, 37, 40, 42, 43, 46
    two-tailed test, 48
average power, 62, 66, 68, 69, 71, 72

B

bootstrap, 147
    lower bound for SP, 147, 148, 153
    estimator of SP, 147, 153
    replications, 153
    technique, 147, 148

C

calibration, 75, 148
chance, xxv, 53
chi-square test
    $2 \times C$ tables, 136
clinical trials, xxii, xxiii, 25
    cost, xxiii, 55, 59, 82, 85
    failure, xxiv–xxvi
      rate of, xxvi
    times, 82, 85
confidence interval, xxviii, 6–8
    for noncentrality parameter, 109
    for the effect size, 8
    one-sided, 8
      for RP, 35
    two-sided, 8
confidence level, 6–8
conservativeness, xxviii
    amount of, xxviii, 37, 70
    optimal amount of, 72, 74, 75
      estimation, 73, 75

Success Probability Estimation with Applications to Clinical Trials, First Edition.
By Daniele De Martini Copyright © 2013 John Wiley & Sons, Inc.

AUTHOR INDEX

Success Probability Estimation with Applications to Clinical Trials, First Edition.
By Daniele De Martini Copyright © 2013 John Wiley & Sons, Inc.